COGNITIVE VISUAL MEMORY IN CATS

ANIMAL SCIENCE, ISSUES AND PROFESSIONS

Primatology: Theories, Methods and Research
Emil Potocki and Juliusz Krasiński (Editors)
2009. ISBN: 978-1-60741-852-8

Animal Genetics
Leopold J. Rechi (Editor)
2009. ISBN: 978-1-60741-844-3

The Animal Feed Question in the Shadow of Contemporary Food Crises
P.E. Zoiopoulos and Eleftherios H. Drosinos
2010. ISBN: 978-1-61668-785-4

Dolphins: Anatomy, Behavior and Threats
Agustin G. Pearce and Lucía M. Correa (Editors)
2010. ISBN: 978-1-60876-849-3

Veterinarian Workforce Role in Defense Against Animal Disease
Justin C. Bennett (Editor)
2010. ISBN: 978-1-60741-656-2

Mycotoxicoses in Animals Economically Important
Edlayne Gonçalez, Joana D'arc Felicio and Simone Aquino (Editors)
2010. ISBN: 978-1-61668-195-1
2010. ISBN: 978-1-61668-904-9 (E-book)

The Integument of Dolphins
Wilfried Meyer
2010. ISBN: 978-1-61668-254-5
2010. ISBN: 978-1-61668-604-8 (E-book)

ANIMAL SCIENCE, ISSUES AND PROFESSIONS

COGNITIVE VISUAL MEMORY IN CATS

V. M. OKUJAVA
AND
T. A. NATISHVILI

Nova Science Publishers, Inc.

New York

For permission to use material from this book please contact us:
Telephone 631-231-7269; Fax 631-231-8175
Web Site: http://www.novapublishers.com

NOTICE TO THE READER

The Publisher has taken reasonable care in the preparation of this book, but makes no expressed or implied warranty of any kind and assumes no responsibility for any errors or omissions. No liability is assumed for incidental or consequential damages in connection with or arising out of information contained in this book. The Publisher shall not be liable for any special, consequential, or exemplary damages resulting, in whole or in part, from the readers' use of, or reliance upon, this material.

Independent verification should be sought for any data, advice or recommendations contained in this book. In addition, no responsibility is assumed by the publisher for any injury and/or damage to persons or property arising from any methods, products, instructions, ideas or otherwise contained in this publication.

This publication is designed to provide accurate and authoritative information with regard to the subject matter covered herein. It is sold with the clear understanding that the Publisher is not engaged in rendering legal or any other professional services. If legal or any other expert assistance is required, the services of a competent person should be sought. FROM A DECLARATION OF PARTICIPANTS JOINTLY ADOPTED BY A COMMITTEE OF THE AMERICAN BAR ASSOCIATION AND A COMMITTEE OF PUBLISHERS.

LIBRARY OF CONGRESS CATALOGING-IN-PUBLICATION DATA

Available upon request.
ISBN: 978-1-61668-293-4

Published by Nova Science Publishers, Inc. † New York

CONTENTS

Preface		ix
Abstract		xi
Chapter 1	Introduction	1
Chapter 2	Nonspatial Visual Recognition Memory in Cats	5
Chapter 3	Spatial Visual Recognition Memory	27
Chapter 4	Two Subsystems of Spatial Visual Memory (Delayed Response Problem)	37
Chapter 5	Conclusion: Memory Revisited – From Retrospective to Perspective	49
References		51
Index		57

PREFACE

The role of cognitive memory in "becoming" of the complexly organized systems is briefly considered from the viewpoint of the general systems theory; the role of Georgian neurophysiologists in emphasizing cognitive aspects of memory role in animal behavior is underlined. The existence of the "one-trial" nonspatial visual recognition memory in cats, as representatives of carnivores with poorly developed vision, is established; it is shown that analogously to primates and rodents in cats the so called rhinal cortex plays a major role in mediating this type of visual cognitive memory. It is shown that in cats, similarly to primates and rodents, parahippocampal cortex (with possible inclusion in this system of the subicular complex) is responsible for visuospatial memory. This new book examines the aspects of cognitive visual memory in cats.

ABSTRACT

This chapter consists of five main parts. In the first one (I - Introduction) the role of cognitive memory in "becoming" of the complexly organized systems is briefly considered from the viewpoint of the general systems theory; the role of Georgian neurophysiologists in emphasizing cognitive aspects of memory role in animal behavior is underlined. In the second part (II - Nonspatial visual recognition memory) the existence of the "one-trial" nonspatial visual recognition memory in cats, as representatives of carnivores with poorly developed vision, is established; it is shown that analogously to primates and rodents in cats the so called rhinal cortex plays a major role in mediating this type of visual cognitive memory. The following part (III - Spatial visual recognition memory) is devoted to spatial visual "one-trial" memory in cats; it is shown that in cats, similarly to primates and rodents, parahippocampal cortex (with possible inclusion in this system of the subicular complex) is responsible for visuospatial memory. In the next to last part of this chapter (IV - Two subsystems of spatial visual memory – delayed response problem) two probable subsystems of visual spatial memory – egocentric and allocentric – are briefly reviewed in the classical delayed response context; it is shown that the first one depends on the prefrontal cortex, while the second one – on the parietal association region. The last part (V - Conclusion) emphasizes authors' persuasion that "mechanisms of recall" from the cognitive memory store might be studied most fruitfully just in the field of cognitive recognition memory because of its controlled nature in appropriate behavioral testing paradigms.

Chapter 1

INTRODUCTION

According to R. Gerard all complex material systems are characterized by three fundamental attributes: 1. Existence, 2. Behavior and 3. Becoming [Gerard, 1961]. "Existence" means simply being of system in the world during some period of time with stable structural-functional characteristics; "behavior" means rapid and reversible functional responses of the system to currently acting stimuli from the environment. Due to that attribute the system after responding to current environmental stimulation returns to its initial state. Last but not least, "becoming" means self-development of the system over time, due to acquisition of individual experiences, accumulation of information about environmental events and self-actions in that environment. At the heart of that fundamental attribute lie some subtle but frequently very stable material changes in the system which remains in it after stimulation. Of course we mean under such changes the engrams, constituting very bases of memory – quite important function of very complex, self-organized systems of different physical origin [Adey, 1967; Ashby, 1960; Von Neumann, 1951].

To-day not only computer scientists and psychologists are interested in the intimate nature and organization of memory system in living brain, but neurophysiologists as well, who possess acute sense that: "there exists a striking break in our knowledge of short-term changes in neural and muscular cells (impulse propagation, synaptic transmission, muscular contraction) and those long-term events in the neural pathways that underlie "memory" and elaboration of new functional links" to quote Bernard Katz [1966]. What might be the reason for such deep interest manifested by "pure" neuroscientists to the problem of memory, which for the prolonged periods of time had been the "promised land" for only speculative psychology and philosophy?

We think that main reason was current success in behavioral science which resulted in the following statement of fundamental importance: behavior of higher vertebrate animals could not be viewed as a simple "chaining" of individually acquired conditioned reflexes (basic principle of "behaviorist" psychology and Pavlov's views of so called "physiology of higher nervous activity") but is determined by some "internal representations" of stimuli perceived earlier in specific surrounding environment. Retrospectively two main opponents of behaviorist concept of animal behavior may be mentioned – psychologist Edward Tolman in USA and neurophysiologist Ivane Beritashvili ("Beritoff" or "Beritov" in Russian, and in Western languages) in Georgia. E. Tolman's ideas about determining the role of the "internal representations of earlier perceived events" in the organization of mammalian behavior are well known all over the world and by this reason we will not accentuate attention on them [Tolman,1932].

Still in 1932 Beritashvili proposed new original concept about animal behavior [Beritov, 1932]. In his view animal behavior in quite new situation is determined not by conditioned reflexes but by "images" of spatial locations of vitally important stimuli. Numerous and diverse experiments convincingly showed that animals (dogs) in the new situation after the first perception of vital stimuli (food or some damaging stimulus) manifest not the chaotic, but directed, expedient behavior. This expediency of behavior is caused by the regulating role of the images of the external situation, which are created with the perception of appropriate objects in it and which are reproduced in the same situation through one or other time interval.

From our point of view extremely important in the concept of I. Beritashvili is not simply the assertion about the presence of concrete images in animals, but the idea about the active role of these reproduced images in the determination of adaptive behavior; in other words, according to I. Beritashvili "images" appear not as the epiphenomenon, but as the active main regulator of the behavior of animals in the new situations.

From the other side, theoretical studies of the forms of behavior in the self-organizing systems, based on the cybernetic ideology showed that as the conceptual construction " the chain of conditioned responses" principally cannot explain the experimentally verified forming of expedient behavior in so-called " emergency situations]", i.e., when system must in a short time be adapted either to the completely new, suddenly prevailing situation or to an abrupt change in the old situation; it turned out that in all these cases system can organize adaptive activity only when it acts not according to the principle of algorithms (" the chains of conditioned reflexes but according to the principle of heuristics (Bernstein N. A. 1966; Bongard M. 1967, Minski M, ; Miller J., Gelenter E., Pribram K. H.,). Biological example of such " emergency situations" can serve the possible encounter of animal with the enemy, when in the very short time it is necessary to make a decision, either about the active avoidance (situation victim - predator), or about the active attack (situation predator - victim) and so forth. In all such cases of "the chain of conditioned reflexes", manufactured in the old situation on the basis of the multiple repetition of the specific behavioral responses under the constant conditions, cannot ensure sufficiently rapid adaptation to situation, i.e. in other words, living organism, acting in the new situation according to the principle of elaboration of the conditioned reflex would perish from the hunger, the thirst, the predator, the chaotic action, or simply inaction faster than would be manufactured corresponding optimum of "the chain of conditioned reflexes", that requires repeated reinforcements of surrounding stimuli with the rewards and subsequent production of the reflexes of the second and higher orders. But in the real life organism frequently is adapted to the new situation quite rapidly "in one trial" , and this is ensured according to experimental data and theoretical ideas of [i]. [Beritashvili] by the precisely descriptive psycho-nervous activity.

This functional role of the image in the behavior is manifested in its motor activity, because of which animal is not simply adapted to the environment (passive balancing with the medium by I. Pavlov), but actively overcomes its obstacles for achievement of the specific goal of behavioral act represented in the images [Beritoff,1965]; see also the general concept of the "physiology of activity" in the work of Bernstein N. A. [1966]. Its "automation" and conditioned-reflex chaining occurs only with the multiple repetition of this behavioral pattern under the constant stable conditions of the surrounding situation and it begins to proceed as a "chain conditioned reflex" [Beritoff, 1965].

The ideas, similar to the above ideas of I. S. Beritashvili were in many respects developed by a Soviet physiologist P. K. Anokhin, according to whom the leading factors, which determine behavior are the "afferent synthesis" and the "acceptor of action" , into which is packed almost the same content, as in the term of "image" [Anokhin, 1979]. Close ideas were advanced by another Soviet physiologist N. A. Bernstein [1966], who on the basis of the detailed experimental and mathematical analysis of the motor activity of animals came to the conclusion that the forming of reaction occurs not according to the principle of "stimulus - response", but according to the continuous corrections according to the principle of feedback. But in that case in the central nervous system unavoidably must exist in the coded form the prior anticipation of the required final result of reaction, i.e. must exist " the model of the required future", since only comparison of the arriving afferent information about the existing situation with that provided by "the model of the required future" can in fact ensure the expediency of motor response [Bernstein, 1966]. In this connection it is interesting to note that this continuous afferent correction according to the principle of feedback is necessary precisely for the realization of behavior, adjusted by images, whereas the automated conditioned-reflex behavior it does not require [Beritov, 1969]. From the other side, the founders of cybernetics, examining behavioral patterns, characteristic for the complexly organized systems, came to the conclusion that one of the "highest" types of behavior, characteristic of animals appears to be "teleological" - the behavior, by which they mean the behavior, allotted by activity, by endeavor and by adjustability according to the principle of feedback [Rosenblueth, Wiener, Bigelow, 1943]. Finally, the "images" of objects moving in the space, which lie at the basis of the capability of animals for the prediction of the future sections of the trajectories of motion, intensively were studied by L.Krushinskiy, who isolated this type of behavior into the group of the so-called " extrapolation reflexes"; it is remarkable, that this type of behavior is achieved " from one trial" that is after the first test, but it is not manufactured according to the principle of the conditioned reflex [Krushinskiy, 1966].

Thus all contemporary data and theoretical concepts of the behavioral science with the obviousness indicate the important role of the "images" of the external world, preserved in the memory, in the organization and regulation of the adaptive behavior of "higher" animals.

Being the students of I. S. Beritashvili, we, naturally paid primary attention to the accentuation of his ideas about the role of "image-driven memory" in the organization of the behavior of animals. Contemporary studies of the visuo-spatial recognition memory in mammals show the possibility of the experimental separation of the engram of " the location of the stimulus in space " ("image of the stimulus spatial location" according to I. S. Beritashvili) to its constituting components - "stimulus" *per se*, irrespective of its spatial location (thus "nonspatial visual memory") and "place" to be remembered *per se*, irrespective of its "content" (thus "spatial visual memory")..

Chapter 2

NONSPATIAL VISUAL RECOGNITION MEMORY IN CATS

As it is well known in experimental psychology the evaluation of memories and their characteristics in people are produced by two basic methods: by the method of "free recall" and by the method of "recognition". As far as we know, for evaluating the memory in animals thus far effectively is used only the second of those methods. Since this part is dedicated particularly to memory in subhuman animals, speech subsequently will concern in essence precisely only the recognition memory, with small exceptions. At the same time we were deeply impressed by the success obtained by neuropsychologists in the USA in the study of recognition memory in animals (mainly in monkeys and rats), especially by the work of M. Mishkin's team at Bethesda laboratory of Neuropsychology.

The selection of cats as experimental animals for investigating the memory of recognition was caused in essence by the following bases: 1. As far as we know the recognition memory was investigated mainly in the primates and rats; therefore it appeared to be interesting to establish its presence or absence in the cats as representatives of carnivores, in particular if we consider the fact that the cat, until now, remains classical object for the neurophysiological studies.

Delayed matching- and nonmatching-to-sample (DMS and DNMS) tasks have been widely used to study one-trial object recognition in monkeys [Gaffan, 1974; Mishkin, Delacour, 1975; Mishkin,1982] and to elucidate the cerebral mechanisms that mediate this type of cognitive visual memory [Mishkin,Murray, 1994; Squire, 1992]. Similar studies have been carried out in rodents [for review see Steckler, Drinkenburg, Sahgal, Aggleton, 1998] and other mammals, such as dogs [Callahan, Ikeda-Douglas, Head, Cotman, Milgram, 2000]. But to our knowledge there are no such reports on cats, although some researchers have shown that cats have good memory for spatial locations as measured by their performance on the classical spatial delayed response task [Beritashvili, 1971; Fletcher, 1965; Konorski1967; Warren, Warren, Akert, 1972]]. The purpose of the present part is twofold – one is to uncover the possibility of normal cats to solve different versions of nonspatial delayed matching- and nonmatching-to-sample tasks and the other – to uncover the possible brain regions perhaps responsible for the nonspatial visual memory in cats.

We believe that the most satisfactory neurobehavioral studies addressing interactions between the brain and behavior have until recently been performed in primates. On the other hand, the preferred study system for purely neurophysiologic studies has to date been the cat. Both fundamental and comparative studies with a wide evolutionary perspective need these two approaches to be integrated. The major point here is that the whole arsenal of state-of-the-art neurophysiologic methods can be used in cats for identification of the basic neuronal mechanisms of recognition memory. With this purpose we elected to study in cats some of the forms of cognitive memory which have been well studied in monkeys. In particular, this relates to visual recognition memory in conditions of one-trial visual recognition, which has previously been studied in the USA [Mishkin, Delacour, 1965; Mishkin, Prockop, Rosvold, 1962] using original methods, i. e., image-based delayed selection. Results of such study already have been presented by us earlier. As regards the cerebral mechanisms of this type of visual memory, Murray, Bachevalier, Mishkin [1989] and Meunier, Bachevallier, Mishkin, Murray [1977] showed that the perirhynal and entorhinal cortical areas in primates together (i. e. the "rhinal area") play the key role in the organization of this type of memory. Is the link between this type of memory and the rhinal area a characteristic of primates or is it more widespread among mammals? As it has been demonstrated by other investigators in dogs [Callahan, Ikeda-Douglas, Head, Cotman, Milgram, 2000] and by us in cats [Okujava, Natishvili, Mishkin, Gurashvili, Chpashvili, Bagashvili, Andronikashvili, Kvernadze, 2005] as representatives of carnivores they can solve the visual nonspatial recognition memory tasks. On the other hand studies in rats have demonstrated not only the existence of visual nonspatial memory, but also the involvement of the rhinal cortical areas in performing the corresponding tasks [Mumby, Pinel, 1997].

In the context of neuropsychological studies of memory, our specific intent was to use the "delayed matching-to-sample" and "delayed nonmatching-to-sample" tests to determine the contribution made by these cortical areas in cats to one-trial non-spatial visual recognition memory.

MATERIALS AND METHODS

Experimental Subjects

Fifteen experimentally naïve adult normal cats of both sexes (eight male, seven female) weighing 3-4.7 kg were used in this study. The animals were housed in individual cages (1.5 x 1.0 x 1.0 m) in which they had free access to water. Food was given once daily, 20 h before testing. Experimental sessions were conducted 5 days per week. The care and use of the animals complied with Georgian regulations, with Guidelines prepared by the Ethics Committee of the Institutional Animal Care and Use Committee of the Research Center for Experimental Neurology, and with the National Institutes of Health Guide for the Care and Use of Laboratory Animals.

Five different tasks were used, two requiring manipulatory responses, and three – locomotor responses

TASK I: M-DMS (MANIPULATORY VARIANT OF DMS). Four cats, two of them males, were trained on this task in modified Wisconsin General Testing Apparatus (WGTA).

Apparatus

The Wisconsin General Testing Apparatus (WGTA) was adapted for use with cats so that they could use their forelimbs to displace objects and retrieve food. The apparatus as described in detail by Okujava, Natishvili, Mishkin, Gurashvili, Chpashvili, Bagashvili, Andronikashvili, Kvernadze [2005] consisted of two main parts (figure 1): A cat start-cage (55cm x 65cm x 60 cm) placed on a table inside a darkened, sound-shielded room; and a test tray containing three identical food wells, each a round glass jar (25 mm deep and 73 mm in diameter), on which different objects (stimuli) may be placed. The stimuli consisted of an array of 600 junk objects, which differed from each other in size, form, texture, and color (the latter providing mainly brightness cues for cats).

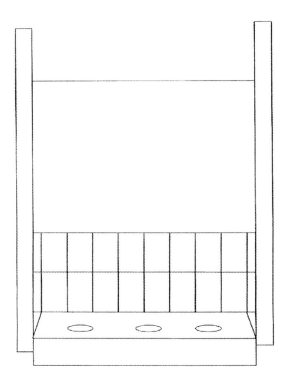

Figure 1. Schematic sketch of the WGTA-type apparatus used for tasks I and II. The side of the cat cage facing the test tray consists of metal bars. The tray, located 15 cm in front of the bars, contains three food wells 15 cm apart (center to center). The opaque screen between the cage and the tray is shown in the raised position.

Procedures

During *preliminary training*, cats were shaped behaviorally to displace cardboard covers placed over the three food wells to obtain rewards (each a small piece of boiled meat, 0.5 cm^3) hidden in the wells. They were then trained in the same way to displace one of three pretraining objects, which were presented singly in random order over one of the three food wells. Finally, the cats were given 20 pseudotrials to familiarize them with the structure of the task: one of the three pretraining objects was presented as the "sample" object over the baited central well; 10 s later the two other objects were presented over the lateral wells, both or neither of which were baited, in random order. The cat was allowed to displace only one of the two "test" objects. The pseudotrials were separated by 30 s intervals. During the 10 s delay intervals and the 30 s intertrial intervals, an opaque screen separated the cat from the test tray. This preliminary training was completed in 7-12 days. *Formal testing* was then begun, using trial-unique objects.

TASK I: M-DMS (MANIPULATORY VARIANT OF DMS) task: each trial consisted of two parts, a sample presentation followed by a choice test (figure 2).

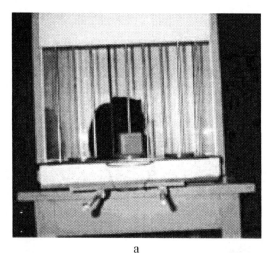

a

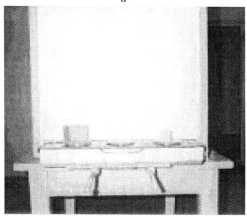

b

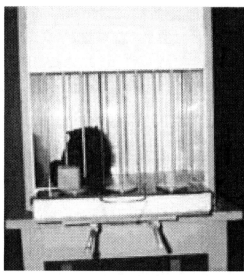

c

Figure 2. Successive stages of the "delayed matching to-sample" (DMS) test procedure is shown below on the photo of the apparatus with cat. A – sample presentation phase; B – delay phase; C – choice phase.

After the animal displaced the sample object from the central well and retrieved the reward (no other object was on the test tray), the opaque screen was lowered for delay intervals of 5 and 10 s in pseudorandom order. The screen was then raised revealing the sample object again together with a novel object, each covering one of two lateral wells, and the cat was allowed to choose. A new pair of objects was used on every trial, and the left-right positions of the sample and novel objects on the choice test varied pseudorandomly. In the choice tests of this task, the sample object was always baited, requiring the animal to learn the rule of delayed matching-to-sample. Twenty such trials, separated by 30 s intertrial intervals, were presented daily until the animal achieved the criterion score of 80 correct trials in 100 across five consecutive sessions. The time limit for the behavioral response was set initially to 10 sec, and to 5 sec at final stages of training; withholding the response beyond that limit was scored as error. The response of the animal toward the central food well was scored as an error. There was no correction for errors, *e.g.* an animal after making an incorrect response to central well was not allowed to correct itself by the response to the side well in the same trial, nor in the following one.

TASK II: M-DNMS (MANIPULATORY VARIANT OF DNMS). Four cats, two of them males, were trained on this task. The procedures were the same as those used for DMS task, except that now the novel object was always baited on the choice test, requiring the animal to learn the rule of delayed nonmatching-to-sample.

Let us turn now to locomotor versions of these recognition memory tasks.

TASK III: L-DMS (LOCOMOTOR VARIANT OF DMS). Four cats, one of them a male, were trained on this task. A schematic representation of the Nencki-type testing room [Konorski, 1967] is shown in figure 3.

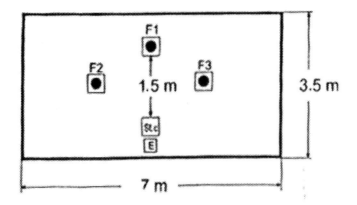

Figure 3. Schematic representation of the Nencki-type testing room used for Tasks III-V. Abbreviations: (St.c) start-cage; (F1, F2, F3) three identical food wells; (E) location of the experimenter. Arrow inside the figure (calibration bar) indicates the approximate distance between the start-cage and the food wells.

The cat cage (labeled as "St.c" in figure 3), measuring 45 cm x 45 cm x 50 cm was equipped with an opaque screen. To facilitate perception of the stimuli from the cat cage, only the stimulus array's larger objects (15-20 cm high and 3-5 cm in diameter) were used in this and following tasks.

The three stages of preliminary training were similar to those given in WGTA, except that the animals were shaped behaviorally to run to the food wells to retrieve rewards, and then to return to the cage and reenter it. The preliminary training was completed on average in 2 days.

Both for the pseudotrials and during formal testing, objects were placed in front of the baited central food well (F1 in figure 3) for the sample presentation, and in front of the lateral wells (F2 and F3 in figure 3) for the choice test. When the animal returned to the cage from the central food well after the sample presentation, the opaque screen was lowered for the delay period (5 s and 10 s in random order, as before), after which it was raised so that the animal could choose between the lateral food wells marked by sample and novel objects. On this task, as in Task I, the food well marked by the sample object was always baited on the choice tests, requiring the animal to learn the rule of matching-to-sample. In all other respects also, the procedures for this task were the same as those used for Task I.

TASK IV: L-DNMS (LOCOMOTOR VARIANT OF DNMS). Three cats, all males, were trained on task IV. All procedures were the same as those used in Task III, except that on the choice tests the novel object was always baited in the case of appropriate response, requiring the animal to learn the rule of nonmatching-to-sample.

TASK V: L-DR (LOCOMOTOR VERSION OF SPATIAL DELAYED RESPONSE). The four cats that had been trained on Task III were transferred to Task V. This task was adapted from the "place trials" of the object-location task described by Parkinson and coauthors [Parkinson, Murray, Mishkin, 1988], in which only spatial location was relevant for successful performance, object quality being irrelevant. For the sample presentation, a trial-unique object was placed in front of one of the three food wells, which were baited, and which the cat approached in order to retrieve the reward. For the choice test, the sample object appeared again in front of the same food well as before, and this food well was also baited as before, while an object identical to the sample appeared in front of one of the other two, unbaited, food wells. The spatial locations of the baited well and of the covered but unbaited well were selected pseudorandomly. In all other respects, this task was the same as Task III (L-DMS).

TESTS WITH EXTENDED DELAYS: TASKS I-IV. Immediately after completing training on the 10 s delay, each cat was retrained to criterion on the same task it has received before, but at a 30 s delay. Two weeks later each cat was tested for retention at the 10 s and 30 s delays, retrained to criterion if necessary, and then trained to criterion at both 5 min and 10 min delays. These tests with extended delays were presented in 20 trial daily sessions in pseudorandom order. Statistical assessments of the behavioral data were performed on the number of trials and errors preceding criterion at each training or retraining stage by Mann-Whitney U test [Hollander, Wolfe, 1973].

For the second subsection of this part only the M-DMS task was used for control and operated cats (bilateral lesions of the "rhinal region"); as general behavioral procedures of M-DMS testing were already outlined above, here we will consider only the surgical methods employed for this subsection. For this reason we performed another study of nonspatial visual recognition memory in new group of 12 adult cats of both genders (seven male, five female), weighing 3-3.5 kg, not previously used in experimental studies. Between experiments, animals were kept in the animal house in individual cages (1.5 x 1.0 x 1.0 m) in which they had free access to water. Food was given once daily, 20 h before testing. Experimental sessions were conducted 5 days per week. Same modified WGTA apparatus was used in this study as already described in preceding section of the Chapter. M-DMS task described previously was used for one-trial nonspatial visual recognition memory testing with all parametric data (trials per experimental day, criterion of performance, delay intervals, intertrial intervals and so on) just identical to previously described.

Surgery

After completion of preliminary training animals were divided into three independent groups each of four cats. In one group animals received lesions to the rhinal (i. e., perirhinal + entorhinal) cortical area (group R, n=4). In the next group, cats underwent all surgical manipulations except for lesioning of the structures of interest (sham-operated animals, SOP, n=4). The last group consisted of non-operated control animals (group C, n=4). All surgery was performed in strictly aseptic conditions on animals under deep Nembutal (40-60 mg/kg) anesthesia. Electrolytic lesions of cortical areas were produced by passing an anodal current of 2-5 mA through an electrode of stainless steel, diameter < 0.2 mm, insulated with epoxy resin throughout its length except the final 0.5 mm at the tip. The coordinates for electrolytic rhinal lesions were selected using a stereotaxic atlas of the cat brain [Reinoso Suarez, 1961]. Cats in the SOP group underwent the same surgical procedures but no current was passed through the electrode. Coagulation of the whole rhinal region was produced by an average of 10-15 insertions of the electrode through small openings (diameter 0.5-1 mm) made in the cat's skull with a drill. Preliminary experiments yielded histological evidence showing that the diameter of the electrolytic lesion of cortical tissue produced by one insertion of the electrode and application of the current with the parameters noted above averaged 3-5 mm (figure 4 ,insert).

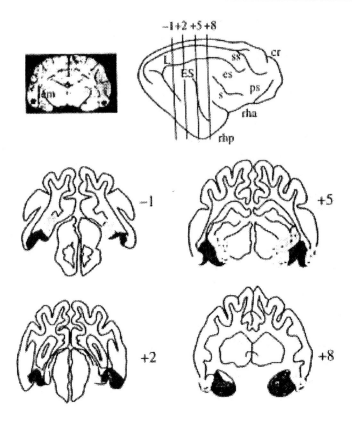

Figure 4. Diagram showing coronal sections through the perirhinal and entorhinal cortical areas of cats with brain lesions. Lesioning target areas are shaded (gray + black areas). Actual lesions are shown in black. The anteroposterior levels of the numbered sections (as per Reinoso-suarez stereotaxic atlas) are shown on the standard scheme of the lateral surface of the cat brain (above right). cr is the cruciatus, es the ectosylvian, L the lateral, ps the presylvian, rha the anterior rhinal, rhp the posterior rhinal, s the sylvian and ss the suprasylvian sulcus. The insert shows a transverse section at coronal level +5, showing the approximate size of the typical electrolytic lesion applied through a single electrode.

After all surgical procedures were completed, the margins of the surgical wound were sutured. The post-operative recovery period lasted 7-10 days, after which testing was started. The borders of the perirhinal and entorhinal cortex are shown in figure 5. By analogy with results obtained previously in other mammals [Krettek, Price, 1977; Witter, Groenewegen, Lopes da Silva, Lohman, 1989], the perirhinal region in cats is presumptively located along the posterior rhinal sulcus, occupying the base and lateral wall of this sulcus (figure 5, A,B).

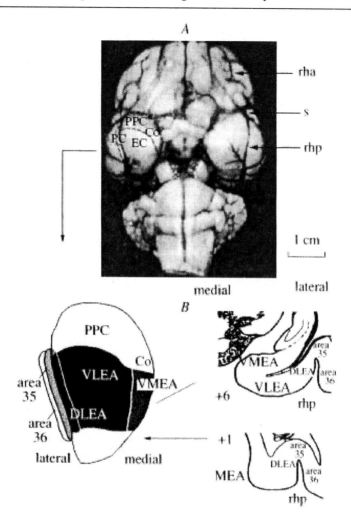

Figure 5. Photograph of the ventral view of a cat brain showing structures of the piriform cortex of the limbic lobe destined to be lesioned. (B) Enlarged diagram of the piriform cortex in the right hemisphere (left side of figure) shows cytoarchitectonic subdivisions of the perirhinal and entorhinal cortical areas. Arrows and diagrams indicate the levels of coronal sections through to be lesioned regions. Abbreviations: 35, 36, Brodmann's subdivisions of piriform cortex; Co, cortical amygdaloid nucleus; DLEA, dorsolateral entorhinal area; EC, entorhinal cortex; MEA, medial entorhinal area; PPC, prepiriform cortex; rha, anterior rhinal sulcus; rhp, posterior rhinal sulcus; s, sylvian sulcus; rs, VLEA, ventrolateral entorhinal area; VMEA, ventromedial entorhinal area.

Its anterior margin lies caudal to the sylvian sulcus (s), where the cortex in the depth of this sulcus is adjacent to the temporal cortex of the posterior composite sulcus. The posterior margin of the perirhinal area is located at the caudal margin of the posterior rhinal sulcus, where the latter splits into the medial-running pararecurrent sulcus [Kreiner, 1971]. The entorhinal cortex (EC) occupies the posterior part of the piriform cortex, which is the ventral part of the limbic lobe. The anterior margin of the entorhinal cortex is adjacent to the prepiriform cortex (PPC) and the cortical amygdaloid nucleus (Co). Laterally, the entorhinal cortex runs to the medial wall of the rhinal sulcus (rhp), where it is adjacent to field 35 of the perirhinal cortex, as medially it reaches the parasubicular area of the hippocampal formation. The posterior margin of the entorhinal area consists of the retrosplenial sulcus, separating the entorhinal cortex from the post- and retrosplenial cortical areas located on the medial surface of the hemisphere.

RESULTS AND DISCUSSION

In present study following results have been obtained:

TASKS I AND II: M-DMS AND M-DNMS.The data gathered on the manipulatory versions of delayed matching and nonmatching are presented in Table 1. The eight cats trained on one or the other of these two tasks learned in an average of 224 trials and 81 errors.

Table 1. Individual scores preceding criterion on manipulatory Tasks I and II (criterion sessions were not included into the trials and errors to criterion indices)

Task I: M-DMS			Task II: M-DNMS		
Cats	Trials	Errors	Cats	Trials	Errors
Alpha	190	66	Anna	180	91
Beta	260	92	George	200	75
Gamma	350	116	Strong	170	50
Delta	220	75	Nancy	220	84
	240	84	MEDIAN	190	80

Although the group trained on DNMS learned slightly more quickly then the group trained on DMS, the difference was not significant. These results differ from those reported in monkeys [Mishkin, Delacour, 1975], which showed a distinct advantage in learning DNMS as compared with DMS. It was concluded from the latter set findings that monkeys have a preference for novelty, a preference that hastened their learning of the nonmatching rule. On the basis of the findings in the present study, it appears that cats either do not have this preference for novelty or do not exhibit it to the same degree as monkeys do.

These conclusions regarding a species difference in preference for novelty and the effects of this preference on learning in cats and monkeys are supported by a direct comparison between the scores of the two species. Comparing our cats with monkeys from Mishkin and Delacour [1975] study it must be noted that in these two cases different learning criteria were used (80% in 100 consecutive trials for cats vs. 90% in 40 consecutive trials for monkeys). From the statistical point of view such comparison at first may seem not to be meaningful. But let us consider the data from Mishkin and Delacour paper: it is evident that their monkeys in M-DMS task ("E-M" in their notation), before reaching 90% criterion, reached criterion of 80% correct responses within 40 trials (median for trials to reach this criterion - 320), after which their learning curve raised monotonously to higher levels of performance (90% correct responses in 40 trials); thus it may be assumed that their monkeys in criterial trials in M-DMS task performed at least as efficiently as our cats in their 100 criterial trials. As to the M-DNMS task ("E-NM" in Mishkin and Delacour notation) monkeys reached criterion of 80% correct responses in at least 60 trials to criterion in spite of non-monotonous character of their learning curve [Mishkin Delacour, 1975; figure 1]. It is worthwhile to mention that according to our results cats after having achieved 80% correct criterion in 100 trials performed subsequent lengthened delay tasks at least at the same (80%) proficiency level in both tasks (Table IV). From these statements one may conclude that it is meaningful to compare our cats with monkeys from Mishkin and Delacour work mentioned above. The eight monkeys in the study by Mishkin and Delacour [1975] learned one or the other version of the two tasks in an average of 225 trials and 85 errors, an overall mean score remarkably similar to that of the eight cats in the present study. However, the monkeys' scores were distributed very differently between the two tasks: DMS, 360 trials and 150 errors; DNMS, 90 trials and 21 errors. As a result, although the cats learned the nonmatching rule significantly more slowly than the monkeys did (two-tailed Mann-Whitney $U_{4,4}=0$, P=0.03, for both trials and errors), they tended to learn the matching rule slightly more quickly than the monkeys, though the difference in this case is not significant.

TASKS III AND IV: L-DMS AND L-DNMS. The results obtained in the Nencki-type testing room are presented in Table 2.

Table 2. Individual scores preceding criterion on locomotor Tasks III and IV (Criterion sessions were not included into the trials and errors to criterion indices)

L-DMS			L-DNMS		
Cats	Trials	Errors	Cats	Trials	Errors
Tetra	1060 (F)	520	#1	510	245
Shava	640	255	#2	725	350
Natsara	900	390	#3	1000 (F)	470
Tsotskhala	1040 (F)	435			

F denotes failure to achieve criterion within 1000 trials. Although two cats (Tetra and Tsotskhala) achieved criterion in additional 60 and 40 trials, respectively, while on the third cat (Natsara) training was disconnected after 1000 trials.

Compared with the cats trained in the WGTA, those trained on the locomotor versions learned relatively slowly, with some animals even failing to reach criterion within the limit of 1 000 trials. The cats in this situation exhibited a strong tendency to return to the central food well on the choice test, suggesting that visuospatial strategies, which are well developed in cats [Warren, 1965; Warren, Warren, Akert, 1972], had interfered with their learning of the object matching and nonmatching rules. To examine how readily cats might learn a locomotor task in which memory for spatial cues was relevant and memory for object cues was irrelevant, we transferred the animals that had been trained on task III to Task V.

TASK V: L-DR. As shown in Table III, all four cats, including the two that had previously failed to learn the locomotor version of delayed object matching, learned the locomotor version of spatial delayed response within just four sessions (i.e., 80 trials).

The results support the suggestion that the cats' strong tendency to use visuospatial strategies in the large testing room interfered with their learning of the object matching and nonmatching rules in that situation.

Table 3. Individual scores preceding criterion on the locomotor spatial memory task, Task V: L-DR (criterion sessions were not included into the trials and errors to criterion indices)

Cats	Trials	Errors
Tetra	60	25
Shava	40	15
Natsara	80	45
Tsotskhala	80	38

PERFORMANCE AT EXTENDED DELAYS: TASKS I-IV. As shown in Table 4, those cats that had mastered object matching and nonmatching up to delays of 10 s committed about the same number of errors as before to master same task at a delay of 30 s.

Table 4. Median errors to criterion for initial learning of Tasks I-IV at 10 s and 30 s, and for relearning after a two-week rest at both 10 s and 30 s and at extended delays of 5 min and 10 min (criterion sessions were not included into the trials and errors to criterion indices)

MEDIAN ERRORS						
Tasks Learning Relearning New learning						
Delays	10 s	30 s	10 s	30 s	5 min	10 min
M-DMS	84	90	0	2	6	2
M-DNMS	80	86	0	0	4	0
L-DMS	413	310	0	4	6	0
L-DNMS	350	325	0	0	4	0

Once they had attained the criterion score at 30 s, however, the cats re-attained this criterion almost immediately both when tested for retention after the two-week rest period and when delays were subsequently increased to 5 min and 10 min.

Previous comparisons of the visual learning and memory abilities of cats and monkeys were based mainly on the use of the learning-set paradigm [Passingham, 1981; Warren, 1965], and these comparisons indicated inferior performance of cats on trial 2, a measure of one-trial memory. Based on the evidence gathered on the tasks used in the present experiment, however, the one-trial memory of cats seems to be quite comparable to that of monkeys, in terms of both overall speed of rule learning, at least in the WGTA, as well as level of retention over long intervals [Mishkin, 1982]. The results suggest that delayed matching- and nonmatching-to-sample are useful measures for investigating the neural basis of "long-term" visual memory in cats. During comparison of cats' performance on the visual recognition task with the performance of monkeys the following distinction is evident: cats perform the locomotor version of the recognition tasks poorly, due to their reliance on visuospatial strategies directed to find food in a particular place visited a bit earlier. Perhaps this distinguishes them, as a group, from monkeys, although this speculative point needs special comparative study. It might be supposed that this difference is caused to a substantial degree by cats' inherent tendencies to exhibit the predatory behavioral patterns directed mostly by visual checks of the spatial locations of relevant objects [Warren, 1965]. These tendencies, of course, should be present in primates too, but to a much lesser extent, because monkeys' manipulatory activity is more developed.

Altogether, it appears that cats, like monkeys, have a highly developed "long-term" visual recognition memory ability. At the same time our already reported results indicate the urgent need to investigate in cats the visuospatial recognition memory *per se,* although first of all, to be logically complete we heed now to report our data concerning possible brain mechanisms responsible to mediation of visual nonspatial memory in cats. Now, our following research step consisted in an attempt to uncover possible brain region sub serving nonspatial visual recognition in cats.

Morphological Monitoring

After behavioral testing, cats were overdosed with barbiturate, perfused via the heart with normal physiological saline followed by aldehyde fixatives. The brain was removed and photographed and cryomicrotome sections were cut; each fifth section was stained with thionine and was covered with a cover slip. Sections were examined histologically. The areas of cell loss and gliosis, along with the extent of the lesions, were superimposed on diagrams of intact coronal sections. Lesioned areas of structures were measured in square millimeters on drawings of each section. Lesion margins were determined using a simple digital system running on computer and subsequent manual calculation of lesion size. The volumes of lesioned tissue in the areas of interest were expressed as percentages of the normal volumes of the areas. The results for each case are presented in Table 5. Lesions to the rhinal area, regarded as combined lesions to the perirhinal and entorhinal areas, were incomplete (mean 75%, range 54-88% for the entorhinal cortex, mean 80%, range 64-89% for the perirhinal cortex). All animals showed some unplanned

Table 5. Extent of damage to medial temporal lobe structures in percents to total volume of corresponding structures

Volume, mm³	HF (406)			Para/Presub (70)			ERh (213)			PRh (233)			Compo (406)		
Cats	Lt	Rt	C	Lt	Rt	C	Lt	Rt	C	Lt	Rt	C	Lt	Rt	C
R. No. 1	0	2	1	61	51	56	98	83	91	56	72	64	6	3	5
R. No. 2	0	0	0	43	57	50	75	83	79	70	90	80	26	20	23
R. No. 3	14	12	13	32	34	33	95	44	70	90	88	89	9	21	25
R. No. 4	9	11	10	51	57	54	85	40	63	92	82	87	29	22	26
Mean	6	6	6	47	50	48	88	63	76	77	83	80	18	17	20

HF, Hippocampal formation; Para/Presub, parasubiculum plus presubiculum; ERh, entorhinal cortex; PRh, perirhinal cortex; Compo, area composita posterior according to Kreiner (1971); Lt, left; Rt, right;

bilateral lesioning of the parasubiculum and presubiculum (mean 48%, range 33-56%; Table 5, figure 4), though unexpected lesioning of other areas outside the rhinal cortex was insignificant.

This included minor bilateral lesioning of the hippocampus itself (mean 6%, range 0-13%) and the area composita (mean 20%, range 5-26%) according to Kreiner's notation (1971), this being unilateral in the latter case – cat R. No. 4 (Table 5, figure 6).

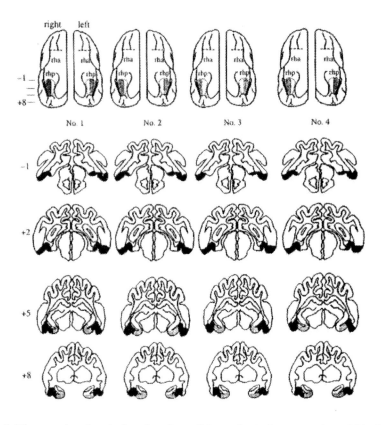

Figure 6. Diagram showing the basal surface of the cat brain (upper row); perirhinal lesions are shown in black, entorhinal lesions in dark grey. Below – reconstructions of perirhinal and entorhinal lesions (black) in four operated cats (R. No1, R. No 2, R. No. 3, and R. No. 4). Anteroposterior levels of numbered sections (as per Reinoso-Suarez stereotaxic atlas) are shown on the standard scheme of the ventral surface of the cat brain (upper diagram). Numbers indicate distances in millimeters from the interaural vertical plane. For further see captions of to figures 4 and 5.

Consequences of Lesioning of the Rhinal Area

Statistical analysis of the results of the behavioral experiments was performed using a computer running the statistical packages Statistica and SPSS 10 (Statsoft Incx., USA). Analysis of the data presented in Table 6 shows that the results obtained from performance of the "delayed matching-to-sample" test by intact and SOP cats could be combined into a single group, termed "control animals".

Table 6. Individual scores preceding criterion (criterion sessions were not included into the errors to criterion indices) in DMS Task tested under "short" (5 sec, 10 sec) delay conditions in normal, sham operated (control animals groups) and operated rhinal cats.(criterion – no more than 20 errors in 100 consecutive trials.

GROUPS:	ANIMALS	DELAYS	
		5 sec	10 sec
NORMAL CONTROL(n=4)	# 1	66	55
	# 2	92	100
	# 3	116	90
	# 4	75	48
SHAM OPERATED CONTROL (n=4)	# 1	102	62
	# 2	69	70
	# 3	75	102
	# 4	100	65
RHINAL OPERATED EXPERIMENTAL (n=4)	# 1	90	120
	# 2	87	110
	# 3	100	130
	# 4	105	150

Single-factor ANOVA demonstrated a statistically significant intergroup difference between control and experimental cats with rhinal lesions to the brain ($F = 5.935$; $p = 0.009$). On the other hand, the same analysis showed that the post hoc Sheffe's test for multiple comparisons identified a significant difference between cats with lesions to the rhinal area and animals of the control group with a 10-sec delay ($p = 0.024$) but not with a 5-sec delay ($p = 0.999$). This is entirely consistent with results obtained from nonparametric analysis and, furthermore, is additional evidence for the absence of any influence of lesions to the rhinal area on the initial "delayed matching-to-sample" training.

It seems appropriate to start the discussion of the data obtained here from the point of view of Mishkin's hypothesis of the hierarchical organization of memory for one-trial perception of objects in primates [Mishkin, Suzuki, Gadian, Vargha-Khadem, 1997]. According to this hypothesis, recognition memory for different sensory modalities (including vision) is organized hierarchically: the hippocampal system receives its main inputs from widely disseminated areas of the neocortex via two main projections - one from the perirhinal and one from the parahippocampal cortex. The first of these projections (the "ventral stream") arises from different sensory modalities important for analysis of stimulus quality, while the latter arises from the neocortical areas important for analysis of stimulus locations (the "dorsal stream"). We will not discuss dorsal stream here in this section as, according to the hypothesis, it is responsible for spatial memory, which was not addressed in the present part of this Chapter. The ventral stream, which is important for the organization of visual nonspatial memory, consists of "higher visual areas" (the inferior temporal cortex) and the perirhinal and entorhinal cortical areas; information is projected from these to the hippocampuses.

This raises the important question: is the ventral stream (or some analog!) present in carnivores? Verification of the existence of such a stream in cats clearly requires knowledge as to whether cats generally have an albeit functional analog (according to the results of Hodos and Campbell [1969] ideology) of the "inferior temporal cortex" in primates. Unfortunately, there are very few data on this important question and these data are contradictory: some investigators have shown the existence of such an analog in cats [Campbell, Jr., 1978; Hara, Cornwell, Warren, Webster, 1974; Natishvili, 1979], while others refute its existence [Gross, 1973]. In general, further investigations are needed to obtain a more strongly grounded interpretation of our data from this point of view. Our data suggest the conclusion that visual recognition in cats is mediated by the same cortical area as in monkeys. It should, however, be emphasized that our conclusion, like the analogous conclusion of American investigators with respect to visual recognition in primates [Murray, Bachevalier, Mishkin, 1989], is restricted only by short-term recognition memory. In our studies, animals of the experimental group (with lesions to the rhinal area) did not differ from controls on testing of recognition with delays shorter then 10 sec. This is evidently further support for the view that visual perception of an object and memory of it (even in the short-term version) depends on different brain structures in mammals. Overall, an important conclusion follows from the present data: visual recognition memory can be regarded as an "evolutionary invariant" in different mammal species. However these species have different ethological and ecological characteristics: it is sufficient to say that monkeys are diurnal, while cats are nocturnal. To summarize obtained results we can make following main inferences: cats trained in the our modified WGTA learned the two tasks at about the same rate, on average, as that reported for monkeys. However, unlike monkeys, whose strong preference for novelty facilitates their learning of the nonmatching rule and retards their learning of the matching rule, the cats learned the two different rules at about the same rate, suggesting that cats do not share the monkey's strong preference for novelty. In contrast to their relatively rapid learning of the manipulatory versions of the two tasks, cats learned the locomotor versions only slowly or even failed to learn. Experimental analysis indicated that a major source of the cats' difficulty on these locomotor versions was interference from a strong tendency in the large testing room to use visuospatial strategies. Thus let us turn now to the study of visuospatial recognition memory in cats.

Chapter 3

SPATIAL VISUAL RECOGNITION MEMORY

Spatial memory, which is studied mainly in terns of delayed responses, is a phenomena which is widespread in different mammalian species [Beritashvili, 1971; Konorski, 1967; Nissen, Riesen, Nowlis, 1938; Olton 1977]. Among the various types of spatial memory, spatial recognition on one-trial perception of objects has only been studied relatively recently because of the development of original methods in Mishkin's laboratory in the USA [Parkinson, Murray, Mishkin, 1988]. Recent observations in primates have shown that the perirhinal cortex, as well as the entorhinal cortex and parahippocampal area, which make up the "medial temporal lobe", play a significant role in organizing the memory system [Mishkin, Suzuki, Gadian, Vargha-Khadem, 1997; Murray, 1992; Squire, Zola-Morgan, 1991; Zola-Morgan, Squire,Rasmus, 1994]. Lesions to the rhinal cortex in primates induce impairments to recognition memory, mainly in the visual and tactile modalities. Unlike early cytoarchitectonic evidence obtained by Brodmann [1909], the current view is that the perirhinal area extends more laterally and caudally along the posterior rhinal sulcus [Murray, Bussey, 1999]. The caudal perirhinal area in primates transitions to the parahippocampal (TF, TH) field, which is presently regarded as a component part of the functional memory system in primates. The analogous cortical areas in rats are fields 35 and 36 along the posterior part of the rhinal sulcus and the so called postrhinal area, located in the posterodorsal direction [Burwell, 2001]. Given the general nature of the cytoarchitectonic characteristics and the nature of the connections, this postrhinal cortex in rats is regarded as a homolog of the TF and TH fields of primates. In dogs, recent neuromorphological studies have shown that an area which is functionally equivalent to the parahippocampal *area* in primates can be found in the most caudal part of the posterior rhinal sulcus [Woznicka, Cosmal 2003]. Considering the extensive similarity in the organization of the brain in felids and canines, we suggested that cats have an area functionally and topographically equivalent to the parahippocampal area of primates (figure 7). On the basis of this suggestion, we report here studies of memory for spatial recognition on one-trial perception of objects in intact cats and cats with lesions to the possible analog of the posterior parahippocampal area in primates.

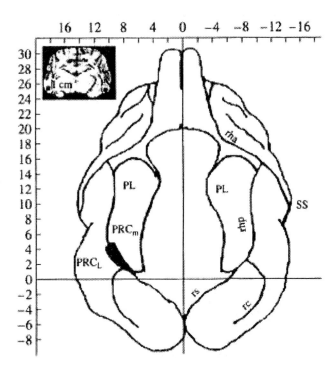

Figure 7. Diagram of the ventral surface of the cat brain. The black and grey areas show the target areas for lesions to the posterior parahippocampal area ["posterior rhinal cortex", as per Woznicka, A; Kosmal, 2003]. Numbers identify the coordinates of brain structures of the cat brain [Jasper, Ajmone-Marsan, 1954] on the ventral surface. PL is the piriform lobe, SS is the sylvian sulcus; rha is the anterior rhinal sulcus; rhp is the posterior rhinal sulcus; PRC_L is the posterior rhinal cortex, lateral part (grey); PRC_m is the posterior rhinal cortex, medial part (black); rc is the recurrent sulcus; rs is the retrosplenial sulcus. The panel at upper left shows a typical lesion produced by electrocoagulation of tissue on passage of a direct current of 2-5 mA through a single electrode.

MATERIALS AND METHODS

Experiments were performed on eight adult cats of both genders, weighing 3-4 kg. Experimental animals were placed in individual cages of size 1.5 x 1.0 x 1.0 m with free access to water. Food was provided daily at 20:00 prior to testing. Experimental sessions were performed for five days per week. Animal utilization and care were in accordance with the regulations and rules of the Ethical Committee for Animal Care and Utilization of the Science Research Center of Experimental Neurology, Republic of Georgia.

A Wisconsin general testing apparatus was used after modification for cats such that they can use the forelimbs to remove objects and obtain food. This apparatus, which has been described in detail in Okujava, Natishvili, Mishkin, Gurashvili, Chpashvili, Bagashvili, Andronikashvili, Kvernadze [2005], consists of two main sections: start cage for cats (60 x 65 x 60 cm) located on the experimental bench in a darkened, sound-proofed room, and a tray bearing three identical feeders, each of which was a round pot (depth 25 mm, diameter 73 mm) on which different objects (stimuli) could be placed. Stimuli consisted of a set of 600 toys of different sizes, shapes, textures and colors.

Behavioral testing of the animals was performed in strict accordance with procedures used in studies of the same questioning primates [Malkova, Mishkin, 2003; Parkinson, Murray, Mishkin, 1988], with occasional exceptions which are identified in the text. The cats were initially trained to use the paw to remove the object covering one of the three feeders. These objects were not used again. Removal of an object from a feeder allowed the animal to see the food hidden within it (pieces of sausage of about 1 cm^3). After the cats had learned to remove the objects covering the feeders with ease, they progressed to formal testing, which consisted of three stages (stages 1–3) preceding a final stage (stage 4). At each stage, each trial consisted of two sequential elements – presentation of the object and its selection. The "delayed sample selection" version of the task was used at stage 1, in which both the position of the feeder and the object covering it served as additional memorization signals. The animal had to use the paw to remove a new object (sample) covering one of the three identical feeders not containing food. The position of the sample above one of the three feeders was randomized for sequential trials. After a 10-sec delay, the animal was presented with the object just presented at the selection phase, in the same position, but now accompanied by another, new object, covering one of the two remaining feeders in random order. The cat received reinforcement in the selection phase when it removed the object seen previously from the feeder in the same position perceived during the sample presentation phase in this trial. At stage 2, the animal perceived a new object covering an unreinforced feeder in the sample presentation phase, as in stage 1, but in this case was presented with the same object in the selection phase – the sample along with its identical copy covering one of the remaining three two feeders in random order. Thus, at this stage only the position of the sample could serve as a relevant stimulus to remind the animal, and it was rewarded when the sample was removed from the appropriate feeder. At each of these two initial stages, the cat received 20 trials on the experimental day, separated by intervals of 15 sec; there were five days of experiments per week and the procedure continued until the learning criterion was reached - a level of 90% correct responses on two sequential days of experiments.

Stage 3 consisted of three subtests, in each of which the sample presentation phase used different combinations of two of the three feeders. We started with the first subtest, in which the presentation phase used feeders 1 and 3, covered by different new objects (subtest "1-3", see Table 7). In this presentation phase of the test, the animal had to use the paw to remove both objects covering the empty feeders 1 and 3.

After a 10-sec delay, the animal was presented with one of the displayed object and its general duplicate in the selection phase of the test, now covering either the same two feeders (i. e., feeders 1 and 3, type 1 tests) or one of the feeders covered in the first phase of the test (either 1 or 3) and the new feeder 2, which was not involved in the presentation phase (type 2 tests). Type 1 tests were tests for the "object-place association, while type 2 tests were simple "place" tests. Thus, in half the tests of this subset, tests were of the "object-place" type, in which the animal could perform correctly only by linking (associating) the object with its feeder place learned in the presentation phase. The other half of the tests were "place" tests, which the animal could solve correctly by remembering either the positions of the two object samples presented or the positions of the feeder not covered by an object in the presentation phase, avoiding this feeder in the selection phase. This procedure gave four different configurations of the tests for each of the three subtests. For clarity, these configurations are illustrated schematically in Table 7. Twelve tests were presented on the experimental day; testing was continued until the animal reached the 90% correct performance criterion in each of the three subtests on each of two sequential experimental days.

Table 7. Diagram representing twelve possible trial configurations in Stage 3 of formal testing. Symbols "A" and "B" represent different stimulus-objects covering respective food wells; on each successive trials different novel objects were used. Symbol "#" represents food wells used. "Plus" sign at the right of object represents rewarded response to it

Phases	Subtest 1 (feeders 1-3)			Subtest 2 (feeders 1		-2)	Subtest 3 (feeders 2-3)		
	A		B	A	B			A	B
Sample presentation phase	#(1)	#(2)	#(3)	#*(1)	#(2)	#(3)	#(0)	#(2)	#(3)
	1)A(+)		A	1)A(+)	A		1)	A(+)	A
Selection phase	#(1)	(2)	#(3)	#(1)	#(2)	#(3)	#(1)	#2)	#(3)
	2)B		B(+)	2)B	B(+)		2)	B	B(+)
	#(1)	#(2)	#(3)	#(1)	#(2)	#(3)	#(1)	#(2)	#(3)
Tests for "place"									
	A		B	A	B			A	B
Sample presentation Phase	#(1)	#(2)	#(3)	#(1)	#(2)	#(3)	#(1)	#(2)	#(3)
	1)A(+)	A		1)A(+)		A	1) A	A(+)	
Selection phase	#(1)	#(2)	#(3)	#(1)	#(2)	#(3)	#(1)	#(2)	#(3)
	2)	B	B(+)	2)	B(+)	B	2)B		B(+)
	#(1)	#(2)	#(3)	#(1)	#(2)	#(3)	#(1)	#(2)	#(3)

Notes. The symbols "A" and "B" designate different stimuli – objects covering the corresponding feeders (1,2,3); new, different objects were used in each sequential trial. The symbol "#" identifies the feeders used ,a "+" to the right of the object shows reinforced reactions to it at the selection phase.

Finally, in the last (fourth) stage, tests consisting of all three third-step subtests were mixed with each other and presented in a random but balanced sequence. In each test session, two different sequences 0f 12 third-step trials were combined with each other such that half of the tests were of the "object-place" type and the other half were of the "place" type. The testing procedure was identical to that at the third stage. Testing was continued for 10 days (five days per week for two weeks); performance assessments averaged over the two weeks was used to evaluate the baseline level of pre-operative performance for each animal. For clarity, these procedures are illustrated schematically in Table 7.

After surgery, animals were tested only in the final (fourth) stage of the test for 30 days (five days per week for six weeks).

At the end of the preliminary training, the animals were randomized to two groups: a control group – all cats underwent surgical manipulations but without passage of the current through brain tissue. Cats of the second group underwent bilateral electrolytic lesioning of brain tissue in the area functionally equivalent to the posterior parahippocampal area in primates (the "postrhinal cortex" as defined by Woznicka & Kosmal [2003]). All operations were performed under deep anesthesia with Nembutal (40-60 mg/kg) in strictly aseptic conditions. Electrolytic lesions in this brain structure were produced by passing anode currents of 2-5 mA via stainless steel electrodes (tip diameter < 0.2 mm) insulated throughout with epoxy lacquer with the exception of a 0.5 mm length at the tip. The stereotaxic coordinates of brain areas subjected to electrolytic lesioning were determined using a stereotaxic atlas of the cat brain [Reinoso-Suarez 1961]. Coagulation of the entire posterior parahippocampal area required insertion of the coagulating electrode at 2-3 different points into the brain through small openings (diameter 0.5-1 mm) drilled into the scull bone with a drill. In the trial experiments histological verification confirmed that the coagulation current parameters used here produced lesions of mean diameter 3-5 mm (see panel in figure 7). After surgery was complete, wounds were closed, animals were given intravenous anti-edema agents and long-acting antibiotics and warmed with a heater. Post-operative testing started after 7-10 days.

After experiments were complete, cats were overdosed with i.p. Nembutal. Brains were perfused transcardially with normal physiological saline containing aldehyde fixatives, removed, photographed, and serial coronal sections of thickness 50 μm were cut on a freezing microtome; each fifth section was stained with thionine and covered with cover slips. Sections were monitored under the microscope to identify cell loss and gliosis and lesion sizes, which were plotted on standard diagrams of coronal sections. The sizes were measured in mm^2 for each section through the lesioned structure, measuring the margins of lesions using a simple digital flatbed system connected to a computer, with subsequent manual determination of lesion area.

RESULTS AND DISCUSSION

Morphological Monitoring of lesions

Brain tissue lesion sizes were expressed as percentages of the total volume of the structure of interest and results for each animal are shown in Table 8

Table 8. Extent of Damage to Structures of Medial Temporal Lobe – Volume (mm^3), Side

Cat	HF (406)			Para/Presub (70)			ERh (213)			PRh (233)			Ph (150)		
	L	R	Mn	L	R	Mn	L	R	Mn	L	R	Mn	L	R	Mn
	0	0	0	61	51	56	28	23	26	26	20	23	75	70	73
	0	0	0	43	57	50	18	25	22	15	30	23	80	75	78
	0	0	0	32	34	33	15	20	18	10	15	13	87	85	86
	0	0	0	51	57	54	10	20	15	30	10	20	90	96	93
	0	0	0	47	50	49	18	22	20	20	19	20	18	17	83

Notes. HF is the hippocampal formation; Para/Presub is the parasubiculum + presubiculum; ERh is the entorhinal cortex; PRh is the perirhinal cortex; Ph is the parahippocampal area as defined in Woznicka & Kosmal (2003); L = left; R = right; Mn = mean.

The data presented in Table 8 show that the posterior parahippocampal area was subjected to a significant level of destruction (mean 83%, range 73-93%) in all operated animals, while the hippocampus itself was not damaged, though significant bilateral involvement was seen in the area of the parasubiculum/presubiculum (mean 49%, range 33-56%, Table 8, Figure 8). The surrounding structures in all cats with parahippocampal damage also showed unintentional lesioning of the entorhinal and perirhinal cortical areas, though the level of this damage was no greater than 40%.

Consequences of Local Lesions to the Parahippocampal Area

These data are presented in Table 9.

Table 9. Pre-operative and post-operative training to perform the "place" and "object-place" tasks in cats with parahippocampal lesions (Ph1-Ph4) and sham-operated cats (SO1-SO$). Eight cats took part in pre-operative training. After they achieved the criterion of performing tests correctly , four cats underwent lesioning of the parahippocampal area and the others served as "sham-operated" controls. For the eight intact cats, the number of trials (T) and errors (E) for achievement of the 90% correct test performances criterion are shown

Cat	Preoperative training		Performance sessions 1-12			Post-operative performance sessions 1-12		
	T	E	OP	P	Mean	OP	P	Mean
Ph1	540	160	72	48	60	120	92	106
Ph2	500	125	60	68	64	98	102	100
Ph3	1220	244	96	100	98	100	82	91
Ph4	460	120	88	84	86	96	100	98
Mean	680	136	79	75	74	104	94	93
SO1	540	135	64	36	40	72	84	67
SO2	620	124	90	104	97	80	44	54
SO3	480	120	90	100	95	94	100	97
SO4	720	240	84	38	53	78	42	58
	590	155	100	70	71	81	68	112

Notes. "Ph" shows bilateral lesions to the parahippocampal area. SO = sham-operated; T = trials; E = errors to achievement of the criterion for pre-operative training including stages 1, 2, and 3. Each column shows the performance, averaged for two test sessions (12 configurations of trials, each including 144 trials) for the "object-place" (OP) and "place" (P) tests and means for the two types of test.

There were no significant differences in performance of the "object-place" or "place" tests throughout pre-operative or post-operative testing in the control sham-operated or experimental animals with lesions to the parahippocampal area (pre-operative, Mann-Whitney U test: m = n = 4, U = 7, p = 0.773, two-tailed; post-operative testing, Mann-Whitney U test: m = n 4, U = 5, p = 0.468, two-tailed). At the same time, a significant deficit in spatial recognition was seen after surgery between the experimental group of cats with parahippocampal lesions and the control group of sham-operated cats on performance of tests for spatial recognition (Mann-Whitney U test: m = n = 4, U = 0, p = 0.02, two tailed). This deficit was apparent to the same extent in the "object-place" and "place" tests.

The data obtained here suggest: 1) that in cats, memory for the recognition of a one-trial perception of associations of the "object-place" type depend on the posterior parahippocampal area; 2) that within this area, both he parahippocampal cortex and the parasubiculum/presubiculum make significant contributions to organizing this type of memory.

Mishkin, Suzuki, Gadian, Vargha-Khadem [1997] suggested that memory for the recognition of different sensory modalities (including visual) is organized hierarchically. The hippocampal system receives its main inputs from widely distributed areas of the neocortical mantle via two main pathways: one running from the perirhinal area and other from the posterior parahippocampal area. The ventral information processing stream, important for organizing visual nonspatial recognition memory, includes the "higher visual areas" (the inferior temporal cortex), the perirhinal area, and the entorhinal cortex at the input to hippocampus itself. On the other hand, the same hypothesis identifies a dorsal information processing stream, providing for the organization of spatial recognition memory. In primates, this includes the inferior parietal cortical lobe and the posterior parahippocampal area at the input to hippocampus. Unfortunately, this question has not as yet been investigated in cats in this context. Thus, there is interest in recent neuromorphological data from cats which indicate that the rostrocaudal axis in the perirhinal cortex corresponds to the transition from the auditory to the visual areas in the temporal associative cortex [Witter, Groenewegen, 2004].

It is interesting to compare our data with Beritashvili's "image memory" concept in higher vertebrates, which is a natural extension of his views on the regulation of behavior in higher vertebrates by images of environmental objects occurring after single-trial perception of these objects [Beritashvili, 1971]. It should be noted that even at the very first phases of development, Beritashvili's concept arose from the following basic considerations: single-trial perception of the location of food in animals is followed by the creation of an image of the food location in the specific situation which can be reproduced after a period of time on repeated perception in the same situation – i.e., both the image of the food itself and the image of its location can be reproduced; it seems natural that the "food-place" association should also be reproduced. The analogy with the views of American investigators (at least in terms of the behavioral-functional aspect of this question) is almost complete. The only differences, from our point of view, relate to the following two points. Firstly, Beritashvili always emphasized the remembering of vitally important objects (such as food) and their locations in a defined situation (which is also remembered but, so to speak, "implicitly"). Secondly, and this is very important, in Beritashvili's studies, as in those of other authors at that time, the experimental data were not subjected to statistical analysis. At the same time, it should be noted that according to Beritashvili's views, only the neocortex is responsible for this type of image memory, while data published by American authors and our own results indicate that this type of cognitive memory is mediated by structures which are less part of neocortex than of the "intermediate cortex", as indicated by Filimonov [1949]

To summarize obtained results we can make following main inferences: 1.Intact cats can learn tests demonstrating recognition memory both for single-trial perception of associations between external objects and their spatial locations and for the single-trial perception of only the position of the object. 2. In cats, recognition memory for single-trial perception of associations of the "object-place" type depends on the posterior parahippocampal area; some contribution to this recognition is also made by the parasubiculum/presubiculum complex, though the concrete role of the latter has yet to be established. 3. Recognition memory for single-trial perception of only the spatial position of an object also depends on the posterior parahippocampal area, with involvement of the parasubiculum/presubiculum complex.

And now to the end of our chapter we want to consider briefly from our point of view the delayed response problem – the problem, from which the original concept of I. Beritashvili about "image-driven" behavior has emerged [Beritoff, 1961]

Chapter 4

TWO SUBSYSTEMS OF SPATIAL VISUAL MEMORY (DELAYED RESPONSE PROBLEM)

Now, let us return to more synthetic aspects of cognitive memory in animals. By "synthetic aspects" we mean here those aspects of memory research, which are closer to its manifestations in "real" life in "real" ecological conditions. Thus we need here to consider more ethological behavior than in artificial laboratory conditions, permitting stricter and more "analytical" research. We suppose in that respect that classical delayed response task introduced about a century ago in comparative psychology by Hunter [1913] might be appropriate for that purpose because at one hand it "models" natural behavior (for instance, food seeking behavior in animals – remember dog, which purposefully seeks the bone, hidden by it some times ago under earth), and on the other hand, in laboratory conditions permits quantitative, parametric analysis of behavior. As we have mentioned repeatedly it is our supposition, that Beritashvili in his memory research widely used such tasks like delayed response for its just mentioned advantages [Okujava, Natishvili 1986]. General logical structure of the delayed response (in its so called "direct version", (see [Fletcher, 1965]) is as follows:

An experimental animal is restricted in the start-cage with a transparent front door. An experimenter shows an animal the small part of food and at the full site of an animal hidden it in one of two (or several) identical foodwells. Just at the same time delay interval starts, after cessation of which an animal is released from the start-cage and its behavior is recorded; if it directly runs to the appropriate foodwell it is allowed to took the reward from it and to return back into the start-cage. This is description of one trial of the test. As a rule few trials per experimental day is given to an animal. Such trials are given to an animal in sufficiently large experimental situation, like those used by Konorski (Konorski, 1970) and Beritashvili (Beritashvili 1971). Figure 9 schematically represents test-situation used by Beritashvili for the study of the delayed responses in dogs and cats.

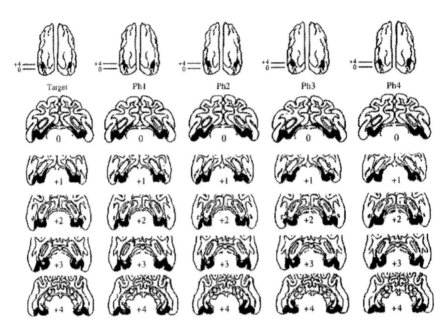

Figure 8. Target lesions of the posterior parahippocampal area (left column, designated "target") and actual lesions in four cats (Ph1-Ph4) are shown on standard coronal sections, which also show reconstructions on the standard ventral brain surface (upper row). Numbers identify the distance (mm) from the interaural vertical plane.

It is important to mention from this schematically view of situation, that it is quite inhomogeneous and reach of external landmarks, which might be used by the animal to localize the goal (food and its spatial location in situation).

How an animal placed in start-cage could spatially localize the food in such situation? Answer is evident – by the use of external landmarks. But this answer has an interesting alternative: what animal would do if situation became quite homogeneous, symmetrical and lacking any landmarks.

As is known from the theory of spatial function there exist two major systems for spatial localization – the egocentric and the allocentric systems (Figure 10).

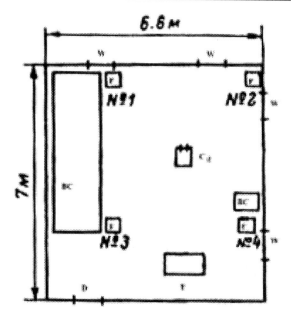

Figure 9. Situation in which all behavioral research of I. Beritashvili proceeded ; memory too was studied in that situation by the delayed response method. Note significantly allocentric (extrapersonal) character of such test-situation. Abbreviations: BC – bookcase, Cg – animal cage, D – door, F – food well, t – experimenter table, w – window.

In the first the spatial location of the stimulus of "interest" is defined in relation to the subjects own location (thus the term "egocentric"), while in the second spatial location of needed stimulus might be defined in relation to external landmarks (thus the term "allocentric"). (Bremner 1982). It is quite evident, that in first system spatial location of the "goal" is completely dependent on the subjects own spatial location (condition, for which the term "egocentic" is quite appropriate, as is the term "personal" system of spatial localization, which is preferred by us in future discussion); on the other hand, in the second system spatial location of the "goal" is in somewhat restricted conditions (see below) independent of subjects own movements (condition for which the term "allocentric" is quite appropriate, as is the term "extrapersonal" spatial localization, which is preferred by us in future discussion).

Now let us consider the delayed response in the context of these two systems of spatial localization. All the following experiments were performed on cats in somewhat artificial test-conditions, modeling in our view the above mentioned systems.

MATERIALS AND METHODS

Experiments were performed on eight adult cats of both genders, weighing 2,8-3,5 kg. Experimental animals were placed in individual cages of size 1.5 x 1.0 x 1.0 m with free access to water. Food was provided daily at 20:00 prior to testing. Experimental sessions were performed for five days per week. Animal utilization and care were in accordance with the regulations and rules of the Ethical Committee for Animal Care and Utilization of the Science Research Center of Experimental Neurology, Republic of Georgia. Experimental situations in which animal testing proceeded were schematically depicted in figure 10.

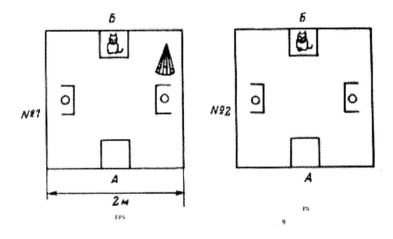

Figure 10. Situations in which our experiments with inverted delayed response proceeded. On the left test-situation to study delayed response in extrapersonal (allocentric) system of stimulus spatial localization (EPS); note the existence of external landmark (pyramid); on the right test-situation to study delayed response in personal (egocentric) system of spatial organization.(PS); note that in that case situation appears to be extremely homogenous and symmetrical, lacking any landmarks.

As can be seen from the right panel of this figure, situation appeared quite homogenous and symmetrical, while in the left panel situation is made asymmetrical by introducing in it of one external object as a landmark. Thus we suppose that testing of the delayed response in the situation represented by the right panel will mean its testing in the "personal system" (PS) of spatial localization, while the same testing in the situation represented by the left panel will mean its testing in the condition of "extrapersonal system" (EPS) of spatial localization. Animal located in its start-cage was shown a small piece of boiled meat (approximately 1 cm^3, or the boiled sausage of the same size) and in the full site of the animal was hidden by the experimenter in one of two identical, symmetrically placed foodwells according to sequences given in Gellerman's table. Twenty trials of the above described type were given per day to animal; testing of the delayed response proceeded until an animal reached criterion of correct responses (at least 18 correct responses in 20 trial daily block). Four cats were firstly tested in delayed response in EPS situation, while after attaining criterion they were tested in Delayed response in the PS situation. Second group of four cats were initially tested in the delayed response in personal system situation and afterwards in the EPS situation. There was no significant difference between these two rules of testing (in terms of both trials and errors to criterion there was not significant difference between the two sequences of testing delayed response: first in EPS system and afterwards in PS system and *vice versa*). But test-situations depicted in figure 10 are, of course, artificial; in real life animals continuously move and thus some kind of monitoring mechanism is needed for both systems of spatial localization.

In order to study this intriguing question in more detail we introduced the concept of the "inverted delayed response" (Natishvili 1978). In this modification of the classical delayed response an animal, sitting in the start-cage visually watches the food, which is hidden by an experimenter in one of two identical and symmetrically placed foodwells, after which delay interval starts. During this interval an animal in the cage was passively transported to a new place, symmetrically located relative to foodwells. After cessation of delay an animal is released from this new place of the start-cage. As is evident from pure imagination, at the moment of release from the start-cage test situation before animals view is a mirror image of situation which existed at the moment of its perception.

Thus, if intact cats were able to solve correctly this "inverted delayed response" task, it will mean that they possess some brain mechanism capable of continuous monitoring of the "inversion procedure" (that is passive transportation during the delay to a new starting point, from which they will be released after cessation of the delay). What kind of sensory information might be used for such monitoring? No doubt, visual and vestibular information might be the only candidates. We have excluded visual information by making the start-cage completely opaque; thus the only source for correction might be the vestibular information. This simple supposition was experimentally documented by us in the following simple experiment, the purpose of which was to induce during passive transportation the highly noisy information in the vestibular feedback system.

Experiments were performed on the same cats used in just preceding experiment with all procedures of testing identical with the exception of the "inversion operation" which consisted in rapid clockwise and anticlockwise rotations of a passively transported animal in opaque cage during some moment of delay interval.. Theoretically one could predict that in PS situation cats will fail to solve correctly this task, while in EPS situation their solving of the task will be deranged, but without complete fail.

Data obtained are shown in the Table 10. One could see with ease from these data that cats in inverted delayed response being tested in the PS situation demonstrated erroneous responses when rotated during inversion operation; it was important that errors in that case were quite predictable in many if not all cases. When vestibular feedback was destroyed by the noise, but memory still existed in experimental subjects an animal's response uncorrected by that feedback oriented it to the foodwells perceived before inversion operation during delay period.

Table 10. Errors in performance of the inverted delayed response (IDR) are shown in normal cats after achievinged criteria level of performance in this task in two situations of spatial localization of stimulus to be remembered – personal system (PS) and extrapersonal system (EPS) under two conditions of testing: normal and with vestibular interference. Errors made in 10 consecutive trials of the IDR are indicated

Cats	Errors in IDR in PS situation	
	Performance at criteria level	Performance after vestibular interference
#1	0	4
#2	2	5
#3	1	6
#4	0	7
Cats	Errors in IDR in EPS situation	
	Performance at criteria level	Performance after vestibular interference
#1	1	3
#2	0	1
#3	0	2
#4	2	3

But what brain structure mediates the delayed response performance in normal animals – representatives of many different species?

Approximately from the pioneering studies of Jacobsen in 30-ties of past century it is well known that quite selective and long-lasting deficit in delayed response arises after prefrontal lesions [Jacobsen, 1935]. This research has induced a lot of neuropsychological studies performed mainly in primates, rodents and carnivores which not only confirmed initial observation of Jacobsen, but led to further delimitations of the critical areas involved in the production of the "frontal lobe syndrome". Because our own research is limited to cats as representatives of carnivores we shall briefly review here the prefrontal cortex of cats and the situation with delayed response.

The definition of the prefrontal cortex as the projection zone of the mediodorsal nucleus of the thalamus is based on the work of Rose and Woolsey [1948] who showed that this nucleus projects to anterior and ventral parts of the brain in nonprimates. Rose and Woolsey however termed this projection zone "orbitofrontal." It seems to have been Akert [1964] for the first time explicitly suggested that this criterion could be used to define homologues of the prefrontal cortex in primates and nonprimates. This allowed the establishment of homologies despite the lack of a granular frontal cortex in nonprimates.

In primates prefrontal cortex is frequently viewed as a "granular frontal cortex" because it contains a lot of small granular cells in one of its cortical layer [Nauta, 1972]. Such layer is completely absent or undeveloped in carnivores and rodents; nevertheless "prefrontal cortex" in those species might be defined if we instead of sufficiently unreliable cytoarchitectonic criteria used other neuromorphological criteria for the percolation of the neocortex in these sub primate species as have been done by Rose, Woolsey, Akert and their followers.

As to behavioral functions of the prefrontal cortex in primates M. Mishkin for delayed alternation and N. Butters for delayed response have shown that with correct performance of the classical delayed response and delayed alternation is precisely connected only small part of the prefrontal cortex – namely s. principalis and within it especially its middle third [Mishkin, 1957; Butters, Pandya, Stein, Rosen, 1972]. On the other hand behavioral studies of the delayed response in carnivores were performed by I. Beritashvili and J. Konorski [Beritashvili, 1971; Konorski, 1967]. Those studies have shown that both in dogs and cats substantial deficits in delayed response performance results following bilateral lesions of gyrus proreus – region in dorsolateral prefrontal cortex in carnivores, functionally analogous to sulcus principalis in primates Having in mind these brief considerations we decided to examine the possible functional role of proreal gyrus in both classical and so called inverted delayed response.

RESULTS AND DISCUSSION

Nine cats were tested in the inverted delayed response in PS system of stimulus spatial localization; among these nine cats six had bilateral parieto-temporal lesions (subpial aspirations) in the middle suprasylvian gyrus, while three cats had bilateral subpial aspirations in the gyrus proreus (figure 11).

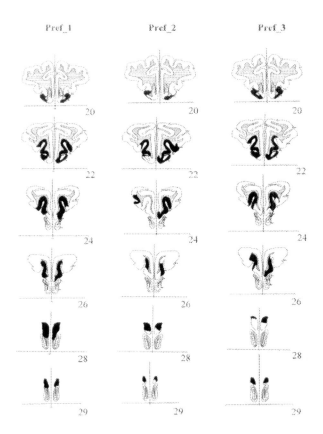

Figure 11. Reconstruction of dorsolateral prefrontal lesions on standard coronal sections in three cats participated in inverted delayed response testing, represented in figure 12. Numbers identify the distance (mm) from vertical interaural plane. Sections are from the stereotaxic atlas of the prefrontal cortex of the cat after H. J. Markowitsch and M. Pritzel [1977].

On the other hand three cats with bilateral proreal lesions and four cats with bilateral lesions of the parieto-temporal lesions were tested in the inverted delayed response in the EPS situation of spatial localization. Twenty trials per experimental day were given to our cats in learning classical and inverted delayed response under two conditions of testing – in PS and EPS situations. Learning in lesioned and normal cats proceeded until their performance reached the criteria level – no more than 2 errors during 20 consecutive trials (one experimental day). Testing situations for the two systems of spatial localization (PS and EPS) was already described above.

Results of these two experiments (performance of inverted delayed response in normal and operated cats in two testing situations are shown in figure 12).

As evident from the data presented in this Figure, cats with prefrontal damage (bilateral lesions of g. proreus) exhibited significant deficits in inverted delayed response in PS system of spatial localization (m=3, n=6, U=0, P=0,01, Mann-Whitney). On the other hand cats with parietal lesions (bilateral lesions of posterior suprasylvian gyrus) exhibited significant deficits in inverted delayed response performance in EPS system of spatial localization. In this context it seems interesting to us to compare our data with the results of American neuropsychologist Pohl [1973], results obtained in monkeys with prefrontal and parietal lesions. He has studied in monkeys quite a different behavioral test – spatial reversals in two testing situations – one symmetrical and homogenous (PS situation) and the other situation with external visual landmarks (EPS situation). Pohl found double dissociation of behavioral deficits in monkeys after prefrontal and parietal lesions: prefrontal monkeys exhibited deficits in spatial reversals in the behavioral situation lacking any landmarks (e.g. PS system), while parietal monkeys were deficient in spatial reversals in behavioral situation with landmarks. These observations are very important because of the following reasons: a) they accentuate the possible linkage of the dorsolateral prefrontal cortex to the "egocentric spatial functions" (although the spatial reversal learning and the classical delayed response task are different behavioral tasks, their linkage to the dorsolateral prefrontal cortex in mammals is highly well documented [e. g. Rosvold, 1972]; b) they point to parietal cortex in monkeys to be responsible for "allocentric spatial function"(although one must be very precautious in postulating functional "analogy" between well-studied parietal cortex in primates and sufficiently less well-studied functions of parietal cortex in carnivores (cats in our case).

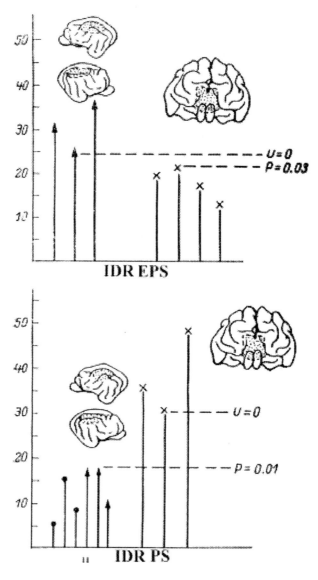

Figure 12. Double dissociation of deficits in inverted delayed response (IDR) in cats after selective lesions of prefrontal and parietal association cortices in the two testing situations (EPS - extrapersonal system vs. PS - personal system of spatial localization) following prefrontal (indicated by crests) vs. parietal lesions (indicated by dashed triangles); dashed circles indicate behavior of sham-operated cats (with ought lesions of the cortical tissue). Mann-Whitney U test for statistical comparisons. Lesion areas are indicated by dots on the cat's dorsolateral cortex.

Now we want to widen our discussion in such a way as to encompass some more general views concerning functions of the prefrontal cortex in mammals. First let us begin with the well-known hypothesis of so called "corollary discharge" developed by Hans-Lukas Teuber [Teuber, 1972]. Briefly speaking according to this hypothesis any self-produced, active volitional movement in the animal is accompanied by such "intracerebral" discharge, which prepares the sensory-perceptual brain systems to those changes in afferent stimulation which will be the result of such movements. Of course in our version of the inverted delayed response start-cage with an animal was passively transported to a new, symmetrically situated place and thus "corollary discharge" could not participate in compensation process needed to "mentally update" initially perceived food well after completion of inversion procedure; in that case vestibular feedback, to our mind, wood be sufficient for such updating. But in "real life", in natural conditions animals move actively and in such cases vestibular feedback functions in parallel with "corollary discharge". In general this brief consideration points to possible links between psychological personality and biology of prefrontal cortex. Interestingly enough from the neuroanatomical and neuropsychological points of view prefrontal cortex appears to be "association cortex" for limbic system of the brain [Nauta 1964, Pribram, 1967] – in other words, the processes mediated by prefrontal cortex of the brain are related to "primitive", simple visceral sensations in such a way as complex perceptual representations (mediated by sensory "association" areas) are related to simple, "primitive" sensations, mediated by primary sensory areas of the brain.

Chapter 5

CONCLUSION: MEMORY REVISITED – FROM RETROSPECTIVE TO PERSPECTIVE

Commonly accepted general model for memory processes includes following phases – registration (encoding of trace), retention and retrieval (decoding of trace); this model works equally well both for procedural (noncognitive, "implicit") and declarative (cognitive, "explicit") memories. Preceding paragraphs of our book illustrated the existence and some neurobehavioral characteristics of cognitive memory in the cat. Unfortunately the deficit of neurophysiologically well- documented direct evidence is yet observed concerning above mentioned separation of different phases in cognitive memory system despite a lot of single-cell recordings from the neurons in the rhinal region and despite the well-documented behavioral and psychological data in support of that separation. We think that major reason of such situation lies in the well-known gap between the "molecular" and "molar" levels (to use D. Hebb's terminology) in the study of memory. To jump successively over such gap one needs, in our opinion, to select such parameter, which will be "macroscopical" and at the same time will in some way reflect the "microstate" of the neural tissue being under consideration. We consider the "slow potentials" recorded from the rhinal cortex to be possible candidate for that purpose. In the course of electrophysiological study we performed recording of slow electric potentials from the cat's rhinal region during different phases of the delay (initial 5 s, middle 5 s and final 5s) in the both DMS and DNMS tasks of visual recognition memory under testing conditions with 15 second delays. Statistical analysis of the data obtained has shown that statistically significant correlation exists between the correct behavioral performance of recognition tasks and appearance of slow potentials in the rhinal region only during last seconds of the delay interval, but not for its initial and middle phases. This result points to the importance of the rhinal region for recall process in the recognition memory (Okujava et al., 2009). Additional although indirect data pointing to the involvement of the rhinal cortex in the cats in retrieval-reproduction process may be inferred from the Table 6 (see II. Nonspatial visual recognition in cats), in which single-factor ANOVA demonstrated a statistically significant intergroup difference between control and experimental cats with rhinal lesions to the brain ($F = 5.935$; $p = 0.009$). On the other hand, the same analysis showed that the post hoc Sheffe's test for multiple comparisons identified a significant difference between cats with lesions to the rhinal area and animals of the control group with a 10-sec delay ($p = 0.024$) but not with a 5-sec delay ($p = 0.999$).

We began this Chapter with brief consideration of the I. Beritashvili's work in the field of animal behavior with stressing his impact in the field of cognitive memory (see Introduction). Now, at the final section we want to ask our reader not to be very critical to our somewhat pretentious attempt to reconsider Beritashvili's "image-driven memory" from more modern position; at least we wanted to fill his theory with strict statistical ground, which he mistakenly discarded. His work reminds us famous Georgian painter Niko Pirosmani, who being an artist-primitivist nevertheless attracts great interest all over the world up to now.

REFERENCES

[1] Adey, WR. Intrinsic organization of cerebral tissue in alerting, orienting and discriminative responses. In: Quarton GC; Melnechuk P, Schmitt F O (Eds.). *Neurosciences – A study program.* New York: Rockefeller Univ. Press; 1967; 615-633.

[2] Akert, K. Comparative anatomy of frontal cortex and thalamofrontal connections. In: Warren, JM, Akert (Eds). *The Frontal Granular Cortex and Behavior.* New York: McGraw-Hill; 1964; 372-397.

[3] Anokhin, PK. Biology and Neurophysiology of the Conditioned Reflex. Moscow: *Nauka;* 1979 (in Russian).

[4] Ashby, WR. Design for a Brain. London: Chapman & Hall Ltd.; 1960.

[5] Beritashvili, IS. Vertebrate Memory, its Characteristics and Origin. New York: Plenum Press; 1971.

[6] Beritov, IS. Individually Acquired Activity of the Central Nervous System. Tiflis: *Gosizdat;* 1932 (in Russian).

[7] Beritoff, IS. Neural Mechanisms of Higher Vertebrate Behavior. Boston: Little, Brown and Company; 1965.

[8] Beritov, IS. Structure and Function of the Cerebral Cortex. Moscow: *Nauka;* 1969 (in Russian).

[9] Bernstein, NA. Descriptions in the Physiology of Motion and Physiology of the Activity. Moscow: *Medicina;* 1966 (in Russian).

[10] Bremner, JG. Egocentric versus allocentric spatial coding in nine-month-old infants: factors influencing the choice of code. *Dev. Psychol.,* 1978, 14, 346-355

[11] Brodmann, K. Vergleichende Localisationslehre der Grosshirnrinde in ihren Prinzipien dargestellt auf Grund des Zellenbaues. Leipzig: J. A. Barth; 1909.

[12] Burwell, RD. Borders and cytoarchitecture of the perirhinal and postrhinal cortices in the rat. *J. Comp. Neurol.*, 2001, 437, 17 – 41.

[13] Butters, N.; Pandya, D., Stein D. Rosen J. A search for the spatial engram within the frontal lobes of monkeys. *Acta Neurobiol. Exp.* 1972, 32, 305-329.

[14] Callahan, H; Ikeda-Douglas, C; Head, E; Cotman, CW; Milgram, W. Development of a protocol for studying object recognition memory in the dog. *Progr. Neuropsychopharmacol. Biol. Psychiat.*, 2000, 24, 693-707.

[15] Campbell, Jr. Deficits in visual learning produced by posterior temporal lesions in cats. *J. Comp. Physiol. Psychol.*, 1978, 92, 45-57.

[16] Filimonov, KN. Comparative Anatomy of the Cerebral Cortex in Mammals: the Paleocortex, the Archicortex, and the Diencephalic Cortex. Moscow: *Medgiz;* 1949 (in Russian).

[17] Fletcher, HJ. The delayed-response problem. In: Schrier AM, Harlow HF, Stolnitz F (Editors). Behavior of Nonhuman Primates. New York: Academic Press; 1965; 129- 169.

[18] Gaffan, D. Recognition impaired and association intact in the memory of monkeys after transaction of the fornix. *J. Comp. Physiol. Psychol.*, 1974, 86, 1100-1109.

[19] Gerard, RW. The fixation of experience. In: Fessard A., Gerard RW, Konorski J. (Eds). Brain Mechanisms and Learning. Oxford: *Blackwell;* 1961, 21-32.

[20] Gross, CG. Visual functions of inferotemporal cortex. In: Jung R. (Ed.). Handbook of Sensory Physiology: V. 7/3B: Central processing of visual information. Berlin: *Springer-Verlag;* 1973, 451-482.

[21] Hara, K; Cornwell, PR, Warren, JM, Webster, IH. Posterior extramarginal cortex and visual learning by cats. *J. Comp. Physiol. Psychol.* 1974, 87, 884-904.

[22] Hodos, W; Campbell, CBG. Scala Naturae: Why there is no theory in comparative psychology. *Psychol. Rev.* 1969: 78, 337-350

[23] Hollander, M; Wolfe, DA. Nonparametric Statistical Methods., New York: *John Willey and Sons*; 1973.

[24] Hunter, WS. The delayed reaction in animals and children. *Animal Behav. Mono.*, 1913, 2, 1-86.

[25] Jacobsen, CF. Studies of cerebral function in primates. I. The function of the frontal association areas in monkeys. *Comp. Psychol. Monogr.*, 1936, 13, 3-60.

[26] Jasper, HH; Ajmone–Marsan, CA. Stereotaxic Atlas of the Diencephalon of the Cat. Ottawa: *Natl. Res.* Council of Canada. 1954.

[27] Katz, B. Nerve, Muscle and Synapse. New York: *McGraw-Hill;* 1966.

[28] Klatzki, RL. Human Memory: Structure and Processes. San Francisco: W. H. Freeman and Co. 1975.

[29] Konorski, J. Integrative Activity of the Brain. Chicago and London: *The University of Chicago Press;* 1967.

[30] Kreiner, J. The neocortex of the cat. *Acta Neurobiol. Exp.,* 1971, 31,151-203.

[31] Krettek, JE; Price JL. Projections from the amygdaloid complex to the cerebral cortex and thalamus in the rat and cat. *J. Comp. Neurol.,* 1977, 172, 687-722.

[32] Krushinskiy, LV. Biological Basis of Rational Activity in Animals. Moscow: Moscow University Press; 1966 (in Russian).

[33] Malkova, L; Mishkin, M. One-trial memory for object-place associations after separate lesions of hippocampus and posterior parahippocampal region in the monkey. *J.Neurosci.,* 2003, 23, 1956-1965.

[34] Meunier, M; Bachevalier; J. Mishkin, M; Murray EA. Effects on visual recognition of combined and separate ablations of the entorhinal and perirhinal cortex in rhesus monkeys. *J. Neurosci.* 1977: 13, 5418-5432.

[35] Markowitsch, HJ; Pritzel M. A stereotaxic atlas of the prefrontal cortex of the cat. *Acta Neurobiol. Exp.,* 1977, 37, 63-81.

[36] Mishkin, M; Delacour, J. An analysis of short-term visual memory in the monkey. *J. Exp Psychol. Anim. Behav. Process.,* 1975, 1, 326-334.

[37] Mishkin, M; Murray EA. Stimulus recognition. *Curr. Opin. Neurobiol.* 1994, 4, 200-206.

[38] Mishkin, M; Prockop, ES, Rosvold, HE. One-trial object-discrimination learning in monkeys with frontal lesions. *J. Comp. Physiol. Psychol.,* 1962, 55, 178-181.

[39] Mishkin, M. A memory system in the monkey. *Philos. Trans. R. Soc. Lond. B Biol. Sci.,* 1982, 298, 85-95.

[40] Mishkin, M. Effects of small frontal lesions on delayed alternation in monkey. *J. Neurophysiology.,* 1957, 20, 615-622.

[41] Mishkin, M; Suzuki, WA, Gadian, DG; Vargha–Khadem F. Hierarchical organization of cognitive memory. *Philos. Trans. R. Soc. Lond. B. Biol. S.* 1997, 352, 1461–1467.

[42] Mumby, DG; Pinel, JPJ. Rhinal cortex lesions and object recognition in rats. *Behav. Neurosci.,* 1997, 108, 11-18.

[43] Murray, EA. Medial temporal lobe structures contributing to recognition memory: The amygdaloid complex *versus* rhinal cortex. In: Aggleton JP (ed). The Amygdala: Neurobiological Aspects of Emotion, Memory and Mental Dysfunction. London: *Wiley-Liss;* 1992; 287–296.

[44] Murray, EA; Bachevalier, J. Mishkin, M. Effects of rhinal cortical lesions on visual recognition memory in rhesus monkeys. *Soc. Neurosci. Abs.,* 1989, 15, 342.

[45] Murray, EA; Bussey, TI. Perceptual–mnemonic functions of the perirhinal cortex. *Trends Cogn. Sci.,* 1999, 3, 142–151.

[46] Natishvili, T. Concerning one modification of the delayed response. *Bulletin of the Georgian Academy of Sciences.* 1979, 93, 161-164 (in Russian).

[47] Natishvili, TA. Some Results of Neuropsychological Study of Animal's Memory. Neurophysiological Bases of Memory. In: Oniani TN (ed), Neirophysiological bases of memory. Tbilisi: *Metsniereba;* 1979, 378-398.

[48] Nauta, WJH. Some efferent connections of the prefrontal cortex in the monkey. In: The Frontal Granular Cortex and Behavior. New York: *McGraw-Hill;* 1964, 397-407.

[49] Nissen, HW; Riesen, AH, Nowlis, V. Delayed response and discrimination learning by chimpanzees. *Journal of Comparative Psychology,* 1938. 26, 361-386.

[50] Okudjava, VM; Natishvili, TA; Gurashvili, TT; Chipashvili, SA; Bagashvili, TI; Andronikashvili, GT; Kvernadze, GG; Gogeshvili, KSh; Okujava, MV. Slow potentials in the rhinal region of the cat brain cortex related to visual recognition memory. Neurophysiology, 2009, 4, 327-335.

[51] Okujava, V; Natishvili, T. On the problem of the behavioral act. *Zh. Vysh. Nerv. Deiat,* 1986, 36, 1156-1167 (in Russian).

[52] Okujava, V; Natishvili, T; Mishkin, M; Gurashvili, T; Chipashvili S; Bagashvili T; Andronikashvili G; Kvernadze G. One-trial visual recognition in cats. *Acta Neurobiol. Exp.,* 2005, 65, 205-212.

[53] Olton, DS. Spatial memory. *Sci. Amer.,* 1977, 236, 82-98.

[54] Parkinson, JK; Murray, EA, Mishkin, M. A selective mnemonic role for the hippocampus in monkeys: memory for the location of objects. *J. Neurosci.* 1988, 8, 4159-4167.

[55] Passingham, RE Primate specialization in brain and intelligence. *Symp. Zool. Soc. Lond.,* 1981, 46, 361-388.

[56] Pohl, W. Dissociation of spatial discrimination deficits following frontal and parietal lesions in monkeys. *J. Comp. Physiol. Psychol.*, 1973, 82, 227-239.

[57] Pribram, K. The limbic systems, efferent control of neural inhibition and behavior. In: Adey W. R. and Tokizane T. (eds). *Progress in Brain Research.* Amsterdam: Elsevier Publishing Co.; 1967, 27, 318-336.

[58] Reinoso-Suarez, F. Topographysches Hirnatles der Katze fur experimental-physiologische Untersuchungen. *Herausgegeben von E. Merck A.g. Darmstadt.*, 1961.

[59] Rose, JE; Woolsey, CN. The orbitofrontal cortex and its connections with the mediodorsal nucleus in rabbit, sheep and cat. *Res. Publ. Assoc. Res. New. Ment. Dis.*, 1948, 27, 210-232.

[60] Rosenblueth, A; Wiener, N, Bigelow J. Behavior, Purpose and Teleology. *Philosophy of Science,* Baltimore, 1943, 10, 18-24

[61] Rosvold, HE; The frontal lobe system: cortical-subcortical interrelatioships. *Acta Neirobiol. Exp.*, 1972, 32, 439-460.

[62] Squire, L R. Declarative and nondeclarative memory: multiple brain systems supporting learning and memory. *J. Cogn. Neurosci.*, 1992, 4, 232-243.

[63] Squire, LR; Zola–Morgan, S. The medial temporal lobe memory system. *Science,* 1991 253, 1380–1386.

[64] Steckler, T; Drinkenburg, WHI, Sahgal, A, Aggleton JP. Recognition memory in rats – I. Concepts and classification. *Prog. Neurobiol.*, 1998, 54, 289-311.

[65] Teuber, H-L. Unity and diversity of frontal lobe functions. *Acta Neurobiol. Exp.*, 1972, 32, 615-656

[66] Tolman, EC. Purposive Behavior in Animals and Men. New York: *Appleton-Century-Crofts,* 1932.

[67] Von Neumann, J. The general and logical theory of automata. In: L. Jeffres (ed). Cerebral Mechanisms in Behavior. New York: *John Wiley and Sons, Inc.;* 1951, 1-31.

[68] Warren, JM; Warren, HB, Akert, K. The behavior of chronic cats with lesions in the frontal association cortex. *Acta Neurobiol. Exp.;* 1972, 32, 361-392.

[69] Warren, JM. Primate learning in comparative perspective In: Schrier AM, Harlow HF, Stollnitz A (eds). Behavior of Nonhuman Primates. New York: Academic Press; 1965; 249-281.

[70] Witter, MP; Groenewegen, HJ. Connections of the parahippocampal cortex in the cat. III. Cortical and thalamic efferents. *J. Comp. Neurol.*, 2004, 252, 1–31.

[71] Witter, MP; Groenewegen, HJ; Lopes da Silva, FH, Lohman, AHM. Functional organization of the extrinsic and intrinsic circuitry of the parahippocampal region. *Prog. Neurobiol.*, 1989, 33, 161-253.

[72] Woznicka, A; Kosmal, A. Cytoarchitecture of the canine perirhinal and postrhinal cortex. *Acta Neurobiol. Exp.*, 2003, 63, 197–209.

[73] Zola–Morgan, S; Squire, LR, Rasmus, NL. Severity of memory impairment in monkeys as function of locus and extent of damage within the medial temporal lobe memory system. *Hippocampus*, 1994, 4, 483–495.

INDEX

A

achievement, 3, 34
adaptation, 3
alternative, 38
anatomy, 51
animals, 2, 3, 4, 5, 7, 11, 13, 18, 20, 24, 25,
    29, 31, 32, 34, 35, 36, 37, 40, 41, 42, 47,
    50, 52
aseptic, 13, 32
automata, 55
automation, 3
avoidance, 3

B

behavior, ix, xi, 1, 2, 3, 4, 6, 35, 36, 37, 46,
    50, 55
brain, 1, 6, 13, 14, 15, 20, 23, 24, 25, 28, 32,
    38, 41, 42, 43, 47, 50, 54, 55
brain structure, 25, 28, 32, 42

C

calibration, 11
candidates, 41
cell, 20, 32, 49
central nervous system, 4
cerebral cortex, 53
cerebral function, 52

children, 52
classification, 55
coagulation, 32
coding, 51
compensation, 47
components, 4
concrete, 2, 36
conditioned response, 2
construction, 2
control, 12, 13, 24, 32, 35, 50, 55
control group, 24, 32, 35, 50
correlation, 49
cortex, ix, xi, 15, 16, 20, 21, 25, 27, 28, 32,
    33, 35, 36, 43, 45, 46, 47, 49, 52, 53, 54,
    55, 56
covering, 10, 29, 30, 31
cues, 8, 18
cytoarchitecture, 52

D

decoding, 49
deficit, 35, 43, 49
definition, 43
destruction, 34
discrimination, 53, 54, 55
discrimination learning, 53, 54
dissociation, 45, 46
diversity, 55
dogs, 2, 6, 27, 38, 43
dorsolateral prefrontal cortex, 43, 45

E

earth, 37
edema, 32
elaboration, 1, 3
electrodes, 32
encoding, 49
entorhinal cortex, 14, 15, 16, 20, 21, 27, 33, 35
environment, 1, 2, 3
extrapolation, 4

F

failure, 18
feedback, 4, 42, 47
fixation, 52
food, 2, 7, 8, 10, 11, 12, 18, 20, 29, 31, 36, 37, 38, 39, 41, 47
free recall, 5
freezing, 32
frontal cortex, 43, 51
frontal lobe, 43, 52, 55

G

groups, 13, 24, 32

H

hemisphere, 16
hippocampus, 23, 34, 35, 53, 54
hypothesis, 24, 35, 47

I

identification, 6
ideology, 2, 25
images, 2, 3, 4, 35
imagination, 41
impairments, 27
inclusion, ix, xi

indices, 16, 18, 19, 24
infants, 51
inferences, 26, 36
information processing, 35
inhibition, 55
initial state, 1
insertion, 13, 32
intelligence, 54
interactions, 6
interference, 26, 42
interval, 2, 37, 41, 42, 50
inversion, 41, 42, 47

L

land, 2
learning, 17, 18, 19, 26, 30, 45, 52, 55
lesions, 12, 13, 14, 20, 23, 24, 25, 28, 32, 34, 35, 38, 43, 44, 45, 46, 50, 52, 53, 54, 55
limbic system, 47, 55
linkage, 45
links, 1, 47
localization, 38, 39, 40, 42, 44, 45, 46
locus, 56

M

males, 7, 11, 12
mammal, 25
mantle, 35
matching-to-sample, 7, 10, 12, 24
measures, 19
meat, 8, 41
median, 17
mediation, 20
memory, ix, xi, 1, 4, 5, 6, 7, 11, 13, 18, 19, 20, 25, 27, 35, 36, 37, 39, 42, 49, 50, 52, 53, 54, 55, 56
memory processes, 49
microscope, 32
microtome, 32
modeling, 39
models, 37

motion, 4
motor activity, 3
movement, 47

N

National Institutes of Health, 7
neocortex, 25, 36, 43, 53
neurons, 49
noise, 42
novelty, 17, 26
nucleus, 15, 16, 43, 55

O

observations, 27, 45
organism, 3

P

parameter, 49
parietal cortex, 45
passive, 3, 41
pathways, 1, 35
percolation, 43
personality, 47
persuasion, xi
physiology, 2, 3
prediction, 4
preference, 17, 26
prefrontal cortex, xi, 43, 44, 45, 47, 53, 54
pretraining, 8
primate, 43
production, 3, 43
program, 51
propagation, 1
protocol, 52
psychologist, 2
psychology, 2, 5, 37, 52

Q

questioning, 29

R

range, 20, 23, 34
recall, xi, 50
recognition, ix, xi, 4, 5, 6, 7, 11, 13, 20, 25, 27, 35, 36, 49, 52, 53, 54
recovery, 14
reflexes, 2, 3, 4
regulation, 4, 35
regulations, 7, 29, 40
reinforcement, 29
reproduction, 50
retention, 12, 19, 49
returns, 1
reversal learning, 45
rewards, 3, 8, 11
right hemisphere, 15
rodents, ix, xi, 6, 43
rotations, 42

S

sample, 5, 7, 8, 9, 10, 11, 12, 19, 29, 30
scores, 16, 17, 18, 19, 24
scull, 32
search, 52
sensations, 47
sensory modalities, 25, 35
separation, 4, 49
sheep, 55
sign, 31
signals, 29
similarity, 28
spatial location, 2, 4, 6, 12, 20, 36, 38, 39
spatial memory, xi, 19, 25, 27
specialization, 54
species, 17, 25, 27, 42, 43
speech, 5
speed, 19
SPSS, 24
stages, 10, 11, 29, 34
steel, 13, 32
stimulus, 2, 4, 11, 25, 30, 31, 39, 40, 42, 44
strategies, 18, 20, 26

students, 4
symbols, 31
synaptic transmission, 1
syndrome, 43
synthesis, 3

T

temporal lobe, 21, 27, 54, 55, 56
test procedure, 10
thalamus, 43, 53
tissue, 13, 20, 28, 32, 46, 49, 51
toys, 29
training, 8, 10, 11, 12, 13, 18, 24, 32, 34
transition, 35
transitions, 27
transportation, 41
transverse section, 14
trial, ix, xi, 3, 4, 5, 6, 7, 9, 10, 12, 13, 19,
    25, 27, 29, 31, 32, 35, 36, 37, 41, 53, 54

U

updating, 47

V

vertebrates, 35
vision, ix, xi, 25
visual area, 25, 35

W

watches, 41
wells, 7, 8, 10, 11, 12, 31
wood, 47